DATE DUE

MY 4 '95		

DEMCO 38-296

Body Parts:

Property Rights and the Ownership of Human Biological Materials

Body Parts:

Property Rights and the Ownership of Human Biological Materials

E. RICHARD GOLD

GEORGETOWN UNIVERSITY PRESS / WASHINGTON, D.C.

Georgetown University Press, Washington, D.C. 20007
© 1996 by Georgetown University Press. All rights reserved.
Printed in the United States of America.
10 9 8 7 6 5 4 3 2 1   1996
THIS VOLUME IS PRINTED ON ACID-FREE OFFSET BOOK PAPER.

Library of Congress Cataloging-in-Publication Data

Gold, E. Richard.
    Body parts : property rights and the ownership of human biological
materials / E. Richard Gold.
        p.   cm.
    Includes index.
    1. Body, Human—Law and legislation—United States.   2. Property—
United States.   3. Personality (Law)—United States.   4. Body,
Human—Moral and ethical aspects.   5. Body, Human—Religious
aspects.   I. Title.
KF465.G65   1996
346.7304—dc20
[347.3064]   96-11852
ISBN 0-87840-617-4 (cloth)

For Trish

Contents

Preface

Systems create their own meanings. Why something is the way it is, as opposed to how, when, or where it is, cannot be answered without reference to the meaning the system has established for itself. If we wish to understand something from the outside—that is, without participating in the meanings it constructs for itself—we can never understand why it is the way it is. Thus, objective observers should not ask why the sky is blue or why elephants have tusks; instead, they must content themselves with explaining how it is that the sky is blue and how it is elephants evolved to have tusks.

Each one of us is not only a biological system, but a more or less coherent narrative of beliefs, conceptions, and hopes. We each determine the meaning of our lives and attach value to the world that we inhabit. To ask why something has meaning for some individual, one must understand the beliefs and conceptions of that individual. When we combine into a society, we carry forward our beliefs and conceptions and share them. We express our shared beliefs and conceptions by the way that we live and the way in which we communicate with one another.

The human body is something about which we have complicated and often conflicting beliefs and conceptions. The body is valuable to us in many and diverse ways, from being the physical form through which we act, to being a source of pride, to being a reflection of God, to being a means through which to express sharing. The human body and its allied good, human health, have been constants throughout the development of our society and are interwoven in complex ways with the way that we understand ourselves and our world.

The advent of biotechnology, and especially its application to the human body in order to increase human health, provides a challenge to the ways in which we have heretofore valued the human body and human health. To understand the nature of this challenge, we must understand why it is that we, in this society, value the human body and what the impact of biotechnology on these values is likely to be.

Because biotechnology results in marketable products, researchers, pharmaceutical companies, and investors will increasingly be making claims to own materials derived from the human body. The way in which these individuals and companies value the body, from a commercial perspective, differs significantly from the ways in which we have traditionally valued the body. These claims by researchers and others will, at some point in the near future, conflict with those of others holding more traditional views of the body. Such a conflict may come about, for example, should a researcher claim the right to purchase an organ or harvest a gene where others would find such commercialism repugnant. These conflicts are likely to be resolved through the legal system since it is unlikely that Congress will intervene in the near enough future to resolve the conflicting claims that will be made in respect of these products of the body.

The legal system, like all systems, contains its own meanings, its own beliefs, and its own conceptions. Let us call the meanings, beliefs, and conceptions of the participants in the legal system relating to claims of rights of the sort that are likely to be put forward by researchers, investors, and pharmaceutical companies, *property discourse*. This discourse comprises the language, norms, and conceptions that will determine who, ultimately, has the right to determine whether materials derived from the body will be treated as a commodity (rather than treated with respect) or consumed (rather than preserved).

This book is my attempt to examine whether, before we are committed to it, this discourse is an appropriate means through which to allocate rights in human biological materials. This discourse has developed during the past 200 or so years to reflect the increasing commercialization of Western society. This discourse is premised, in large measure, on the conceptions and norms of the market. Given that the body and materials derived from it have, since the abolition of slavery, been exempt from these market norms, it may not be wise to apply property discourse to the resolution of disputes relating to the body and its materials. Before the courts determine that materials derived from the body are property, we have time to consider whether there is some better way than through property discourse to balance the concerns voiced by researchers, pharmaceutical companies, investors, patients, and others.

The application of property discourse to the body and related materials involves the superimposition of one system (property discourse, complete with its own set of meanings) on another (our ways of valuing the human body, complete with the meanings that we attach to the body). Here one system of meaning, property discourse, determines which meanings that we attach to the body will be given voice through the allocation of rights to the body and related material. To the extent that there are differences between these two systems of meaning, we must find ways to bridge them or to decide which system ought to be paramount.

This book is divided into two main parts. In the first part, corresponding roughly to chapters 2 through 6, I examine property discourse and the meanings that are important within it. Specifically, I analyze several series of court decisions to determine the bases upon which property rights are allocated. While the decisions of courts may often seem distant from everyday life, court decisions relating to the allocation of property rights are different. This is so because property rights are rights that individuals have against everyone else in society and include not only such negative rights as not to be bothered or interfered with, but also such positive rights as the right to use, to consume, and to sell the subject matter of that right. In this way, court decisions regarding property rights determine which goods we are entitled to use in our daily lives. My analysis in these chapters has led me to conclude that property rights are awarded on the basis of the values that we generally associate with the market.

In the second part, corresponding roughly to chapters 1 and 7 through 9, I analyze the system of meaning that we attach to the human body and human health, and ask whether this system is compatible with property discourse. Because I find that the body has traditionally been and continues to be valued in many ways (such as respect, dignity, community, and sharing) that we do not normally associate with the market, I conclude that the application of property discourse to the body and related materials will lead us to make decisions about these materials based on market norms rather than the systems of meanings that we currently attach to the body and its related materials.

For those interested primarily in legal analysis of property law and the values implicit in it, I suggest reading chapters 2 through 6. For those more interested in the philosophy of value, I suggest reading chapters 1 and 7 through 8. For those whose main area of interest is practical reason, I suggest reading chapters 1, 2, 8 and 9. While each chapter is fairly self-contained, chapters 3 through 6 are best read in their current order as they build to some degree upon one another. In any event, I recommend reading chapter 1, as it provides an overview of the argument against the application of property discourse to the allocation of rights to human biological materials.

I gratefully acknowledge the financial assistance of the Social Sciences and Humanities Research Council of Canada, the Mackenzie King Foundation, and the University of Michigan with respect to the research and preparation of this book. I wish to thank Tory Tory DesLauriers & Binnington for permitting me the time to edit this book and for the use of their facilities in writing this book. Parts of this book were previously published in the San Diego Law Review.

This book was written in partial fulfillment of the requirements for the grant of an S.J.D. at the University of Michigan Law School.

As no book is the creation of just one person, despite the fact that only the author's name attaches to the work, I wish to thank those individuals who made this book possible. These individuals are not only partially responsible for the existence of this book, but significantly improved it by their efforts, despite my failure to always heed their advice. Of all those who provided suggestions, comments, support, and fellowship during the preparation of this book, I particularly wish to thank the following: Patricia Delaney, who not only provided joy and support, but suggested that the *Moore* case provided an excellent basis for a thesis; Jack and Sylvia Gold, for their support and seeing me through my many years of schooling; David Foulds, who graciously provided editorial and research assistance; John Samples, Director of Georgetown University Press, for helping make this book more accessible to a social science audience; James B. White, William Miller, Elizabeth Anderson, and Mayo Moran, with whom I discussed various aspects of this book and who commented on early drafts of this book; and my S.J.D. thesis panel, Heidi Li Feldman,

Christina Whitman, and my supervisor, Rebecca Eisenberg. As for creative inspiration, I could not have written much of this book without the music of Mary Black, Annie Lennox, June Tabor, and Lucinda Williams playing in the background.

1

The Diversity of Values

. . . and to ask gently, but in all sincerity, the ever-recurring query of the ages, Is not life more than meat, and the body more than raiment?[1]

The human body is recognizably valuable. We value the body as a representation of our external existence, as being beautiful, as an object of longing, as providing comfort, and as the form with which and against which we measure and understand the world. Not all of the ways we value the body are universally appropriate, and some of these ways are never suitable. For example, it is no longer appropriate, in this society, to value a human body as a source of slave labor, nor is it always appropriate to value a body in terms of warmth or comfort.

Not only do we value the human body in diverse ways, but in carrying out our different roles within society—for example, as lover or as supervisor—we value the body differently at different times and in different settings. I value my body in one way when I exercise and in quite a different way when I visit my doctor. And just as one values one's own body diversely at different times, one values the bodies of others distinctly in distinct settings and dissimilarly from the way one values one's own body.

The advent and success of the biological sciences of genetics and microbiology and the technologies falling under the general heading of biotechnology[2] expand and challenge the ways in which we value the human body. Through biotechnology we can extract and manipulate cells, proteins, and DNA[3] to form new biological forms and pharmaceutical products that we value as objects of curiosity, as the building blocks of more research, or as integral components of human health. Along with providing these additional ways of valuing the body, these sciences and technologies challenge traditional ways of

1

valuing the body—as, for example, a sacred whole or an immutable object.

The impact of biotechnology on the way we value the human body is not limited to simply causing us to recalibrate the ways in which we value the body; the advent of biotechnology creates a setting in which to value the body and its components as commodities. The products of biotechnology from genetic therapies, to hormones, to pharmaceuticals are things that we buy, sell, and trade. The body itself, when understood as the mine from which we extract these products, is similarly valuable as a commodity. There is a tension, however, between valuing the body and its components as commodities and valuing them in terms of warmth, identity, and comfort. Unlike pharmaceuticals, we cannot buy or sell warmth and friendship without doing serious injury to what we mean by those terms.

My aim in this book is to examine how we, in our society, can hope to cope and resolve this tension between valuing the human body and its components as commodities and valuing them in more traditional ways. This resolution is necessary if we wish both to reap the benefits of biotechnology—in terms of better health—and to preserve the many ways in which we currently value the human body. Whether and to what extent this resolution will be successful depends, in large measure, on how, to whom, and for which purposes society grants the right to make decisions about the human body and its components.

One of the primary ways in which society allocates rights to make decisions about things is through the law, specifically the law relating to property.[4] A property right is no more and no less than the right to make certain decisions about things, from the right to use, to the right to sell, to the right to destroy that thing. Property rights are both positive, in that they represent society's sanction to do something—such as to consume or to destroy a thing—and negative, in that they permit the holder of the right to prevent others from doing something—such as using or touching a thing. To have a property right to the body or to a component of the body is to have the power to make decisions about the fate and use of the body or component.

While property rights were once conceived to provide the holder of those rights with absolute dominion over the subject matter of those rights—one could grow what one wanted, manufacture what one wanted, and invite whomsoever one wanted on one's land—

property rights, as currently conceived, are subject to myriad restrictions—one cannot produce noxious fumes on one's land, build a structure on one's land without a permit, or make loud noises on one's land. Nevertheless, the historical conception of property as providing a space of absolute dominion continues to inform many of the ways in which we discuss property rights and provides a psychological hurdle one must traverse before one restricts a property right for the sake of another right, such as a right to equality or a right to free speech.

Property rights are rights that members of society have against each other. For example, it is no good for me to claim ownership of a pen against the demands of a martian because the martian does not live by and under the rules imposed by our society. The pen is an instantiation of a norm—the exclusive rights of use and possession—that we, as members of this society at this time, have agreed or acquiesced in following. When we grant property rights to each other—assuming that we grant rights for certain nonarbitrary reasons—we do so on the basis of one or more ways of valuing the object or the individual to whom we grant the rights. That is, the determination of who should get which rights to which object depends on how we, in society, value the object—as beautiful, as a luxury, or as a commodity—and the recipient of the right—as deserving, as having highly developed tastes, or as a consumer.

Ways of valuing things are similarly products of our society and the circumstances that constitute living within that society. Therefore, gifts mean nothing in the absence of other people to whom to give these gifts, and they mean different things in different cultures. A gift may be valued in one culture as demonstrating concern or love, in another as sharing, and in still another as establishing a reciprocal obligation to give. The ways in which we value things—call them *modes of valuation*—are both socially and circumstantially contingent.

If, as I have argued, both property rights and modes of valuation are contingent on society and the circumstances existing within that society, then the superimposition of one of these, property, on the second, modes of valuation, must necessarily also be socially contingent. Through property law, we grant certain individuals the right to make decisions about particular objects; we do so on the basis of socially contingent ways of valuing that object and that individual, whatever these happen to be. Since the object to which property rights attach is itself valuable in certain socially contingent ways, in allocating property rights to that object, we effectively give control over the object to that individual who values it in a manner that we find valuable. In other words, the person to whom we grant property rights must either be valuable in her or himself or she or he must value (based on her or his own mode of valuation) the good in a valuable (based on our mode of valuation when allocating property rights) manner. The result of this superimposition of one mode of valuation (that inherent in property law) upon the other (the way individuals value things) is that only certain modes of valuing things will result in the allocation of property rights.

Whether we grant rights in an object to individuals because of the way that they value the object, because of the kind of individuals they are—in terms of fulfilling a particular role within society, such as researcher, entrepreneur, or patient—or because we value something they have accomplished—for example, they discovered a new drug, they made people laugh, or they gave good advice—we are granting the right to make decisions about the object to individuals who value the object in accordance with only a subset of all the possible ways of valuing that object. Consider, for example, one individual who admires the beauty of the ocean, complete with its fauna and flora, and another who values the ocean for the fish he or she can catch and sell. We do not grant property rights to the sea, so we do not grant any rights to the first individual. We do, however, grant fishing licenses that are available to the second individual. We therefore empower the second individual to follow through on the way he or she values the ocean—as a source of fish to sell—but we do not similarly empower the first individual to follow through on his or her method of valuing the sea—as a source of beauty. Call the effect of granting rights of control to the second individual as *encouraging* that individual's way of valuing the body. Conversely, call the effect of granting to others rights of control over an object as *discouraging* one's own mode of valuation since one's mode of valuation is subordinate, given that one does not have control, to the mode of valuation held by the individual having control.

When we, through society, grant rights to make decisions about the human body and its components to individuals carrying out a particular role within society, we give them the power to enforce their way of valuing the body and its components against others who have no such rights. Since the ways these selected individuals value the body and its components are not random—we, through property law, selected these individuals because of the way that we value them or the objects they value—we encourage those modes of valuation held by this select group and discourage the modes of valuation held by others.

Notice also that it matters little whether we allocate rights of control on the basis of how the individual to whom rights are allocated values the good or on the basis of the value of that individual her or himself. In the first case, we, through property discourse, are selecting favored modes of valuation in the decision to allocate rights. But unless we are willing to grant rights based on such reasoning as "person A is valuable, therefore person A is entitled to have a property right in anything of A's choosing" (that is, without there being a nexus between the good being allocated and the reason why we value the individual), the decision to allocate a good to a valuable person must be based on how that person is likely to control the good. We therefore allocate the good on the basis of the role the individual plays within society—the person will cherish it or conduct research on it—or because the good—such as a prize or gold medal—symbolizes the value of the individual. Either way, all of us, including the individual, understand that the good is being allocated to her or him because of what she or he is expected to do with it. Although nothing forces the individual not to use or value the good in some other way, the social expectation will generally dictate how the individual will value the good in practice.

The result of the interaction between property law and the body is that, through the allocation of rights of control, society implicitly sanctions certain modes of valuing the human body and its materials, and discourages others. Which modes of valuation are encouraged and which are discouraged depends largely on which modes of valuing the body we, through property law, are likely to select—by allocating rights of control to those individuals who value the human body in exactly that way—and which will be left behind. Before biotechnology irrevocably sets us down the path of applying property law to the human body, its components, and its derivative products—or *human biological materials*[5]—we have the opportunity to examine whether we wish to accept the modes of valuation that property law implies.

Discourse and the Law

Property law is a product of social interaction. What property means to us today is vastly different from what it meant several hundred years ago.[6] In feudal times property represented a web of obligations, not only between king and lord and between lord and villein but between husband and wife and father and children. While the villein owed payment in terms of crops, labor, and defense to the lord and the lord owed the same to the king, the king owed protection and justice to the lord, and the lord owed protection and justice to the villein.

In addition to landholders themselves, the families of these landholders also had strong claims to the land. A husband or wife had the right, in certain circumstances, not to be deprived of the use of the land at the death of their spouse, and children had the right to inherit the land. Thus, landholders did not possess the right to sell land since the landholder only had the right to control the land during his[7] lifetime and even then only subject to the obligations to king, family, and villein.

With the rise of the bourgeoisie, the inherent obligations to others that had been a component of property law gradually loosened until, today, each aspect of ownership, from the right to use, to the right to possess, to the right to sell, to the right to inherit, are separable and can be possessed by different individuals.[8] What was once a web of obligations and rights is now a bundle of rights that can be unbundled and parceled out in bits and pieces.

While we continue to describe the rights to use and control things as property, as illustrated, the understanding of what that term means has significantly transformed over the past several hundred years. The conception of property law, and the vocabulary and assumptions used to explicate that conception, held by those who applied and used it several hundred years ago is dramatically different from the conception and the associated vocabulary and assumptions held by contemporary judges and lawyers. In this book, I undertake to elucidate the contemporary conception of property law. This conception, together with the assumptions and the language used by those who apply and use it, is what I call *property discourse*. I will also examine how that discourse influences which modes of valuing the body we, through the application of this discourse, are likely to encourage and which we are likely to discourage.

The property discourse that counts, in the sense of affecting the allocation of rights of control over the human body and its components, is the discourse undertaken by judges, lawyers, and legislators. While others may talk about property and may even possess a sophisticated conception of property, their discussion of property law will not, at least directly, influence property discourse. This is because, within our society, the sources of legitimate interpretation of the law are limited to texts, modes of analysis, and individuals sanctioned by society. The law of property is, therefore, what the courts, lawyers, and legislators say it is, even if others do not share their view. Here a distinction must be drawn between the law as it is and as it ought to be. The question of what the law ought to be is a question for political or moral theory, while the question of what the law is falls within the exclusive domain of those sanctioned by society to explicate the law: judges, lawyers, and legislators. The two need not be the same.

Property discourse then is the sum of the assumptions, conceptions, and language used by judges, lawyers, and legislators in allocating rights of control over goods. For there to be anything that we may consistently refer to as property discourse, there must be a minimum consensus of which assumptions, conceptions, and language count in making arguments for or against the allocation of property rights.

By examining the nature of legitimate legal sources, we can see how this consensus is created. There are two facts about legitimate sources of law that support this proposition.[9] First, legal sources are historical. These include treatises on the law, including eighteenth and nineteenth century works, congressional debates, and, most significantly in common-law systems such as the United States, court decisions from past cases. Second, in any sophisticated legal system, the quantity of information, thoughts, judgments, and rules contained in those sources far surpasses the ability of any one or group of individuals to fully comprehend. Judges, lawyers, and legislators, the legitimate explicators of the law, can realistically grasp only a small portion of these sources and their content and will only hold a general understanding of the remainder. Because lawyers within a particular field tend to do the same type of work, the areas in which they hold specialized and detailed knowledge of legal sources and the areas in respect of which they hold only a general knowledge of the law are relatively consistent from practitioner to practitioner.

Because a practitioner practicing in a particular area of the law has detailed knowledge of the range of sources touching on that area and appreciates the often-conflicting assumptions and conceptions within those sources, the practitioner will ascribe few strong principles—of the type, in fact situation X, the legal result is Y—and many weak principles—of the form, fact situations of the type X tend to lead to legal conclusion Y—to that specialized area of law. On the other hand, holding only a general knowledge of all other areas of the law, the practitioner has far less appreciation for the subtleties in those areas of law. The practitioner is, therefore, more likely to understand these nonspecialized areas in terms of a significantly higher proportion of strong principles compared with weak principles.

Legal practitioners tend to practice in common areas of the law, given that they generally serve the same communities. Whether general practitioners or specialists, practitioners focus on particular, practical questions within the law and rarely deal with the theories underpinning that area of practice. For example, an attorney who possesses extensive knowledge of the law relating to whether an employer may require an employee not to compete with the employer is unlikely to have detailed knowledge of political theory or welfare economics as applied to the employer–employee relationship. In other words, the areas of legal practice in which practitioners have extensive knowledge—and thus possess a full appreciation of the complexities, conceptions, and assumptions relating to those areas—are relatively narrow and of a practical, as opposed to a theoretical, nature.

The result of the existence of these shared, narrow areas of knowledge within a larger legal system in which most practitioners have only a general understanding is that, to most practitioners, the law consists of many strong principles, especially where theoretical issues are implicated, and fewer weaker principles falling within the practitioner's particular areas of expert knowledge. Since practitioners do not, generally, travel the seas of generality, preferring to remain on their islands of understanding, the law appears to them as possessing many strong principles even though, if one were to examine the sources of law relating to those principles in detail, one would find as much subtlety as the practitioners find in their own particular areas of practice.

It is the generality with which legal practitioners view most of the law that provides the opportunity for consistent and stable discourse within the law. The strong principles through which practitioners understand the vast proportion of the law provide the basis for the assumptions and conceptions that underlie discourse. These assumptions and conceptions go unnoticed in property discourse just because they are the shared assumptions and conceptions of those participating in that discourse. While there is nothing, in principle, from deterring any individual lawyer, judge, or legislator from questioning these assumptions or conceptions, the opportunity for doing so is seldom provided. The daily task of practicing law generally shoves aside deep theoretical questions; on those few occasions where practitioners challenge these assumptions, they often dramatically change the law.

The assumptions and conceptions underlying property discourse affect not only the discourse itself, but the allocation of property rights made using that discourse, through their influence on how that discourse is carried out. This is especially so where the assumptions and conceptions touch on the theory underlying the allocation of rights. By assuming away theoretical concerns based on accepted— in the sense of being the subject of a strong principle—conceptions of property, legal practitioners are led, without examination, to certain results rather than to others. This has its effects on which modes of valuation are ultimately encouraged through the award of property rights. If property discourse affects the allocation of rights of control and the grant of rights of control encourages certain, but not other, modes of valuation, property discourse itself leads to the encouragement of certain modes of valuation over others.

Goods and Value

One of the theses of this book is that property discourse carries with it the assumption that those things that are subject to it—that is, things that are the property of someone—are best allocated through the market. This assumption has three components. The first of these is that different objects are valuable to us, and ought to be distributed, according to different modes of valuation. The second component is that, whatever these different modes of valuation are, they can be translated into or thought of in terms of a market price. Third, the market will allocate the object in accordance with the most significant of these modes of valuation, using market price as a guide. That is, an object may be valuable to different people for different reasons. When individuals decide how much to spend to purchase that object, they translate the way they value the object into a money price. The person who values the object most will attribute the highest price to it and will, through the auspices of the market, come to own the object. Thus the object ends up in the hands of the person who most valued it.

Although, as discussed, property rights are rights against other people, they are about things in the world. These things may be tangible, such as a chair or a clock, or intangible, such as friendship or the right to copy a painting. Things may be valuable to someone in accordance with one or more authentic modes of valuation. An authentic mode of valuation is one in accordance with which, in a given society, it is rational to value the thing.[10] Only by valuing things in accordance with authentic modes of valuation does the mode of valuation have any social meaning. One cannot demonstrate love, friendship, or hate, for example, to another outside of a society in which love, friendship, and hate have social meanings. Similarly, valuing an historic building or a beautiful landscape only has meaning to others—and thus is rational—within a society that admires things for their historic connection or beauty.

To the extent that things contribute to the good life—a life in which things are appropriately and authentically valued—they are *goods*. A good differs from a bare thing in that a good must be valuable in accordance with some authentic mode of valuation, while a thing need not be valuable. Friendship, comfort, money, food, and luxuries are all goods, but so are, in the right circumstances, hate and greed. Murder and villainy are less likely candidates for goodness, but society has always found ways to value them—such as killing an enemy or betraying thieves.

A particular good may be valuable for different reasons. A piece of chalk, for example, is valuable as a writing instrument, in assisting one to measure clothing, and for its color. It is of negative value in that it squeaks on chalkboards and it leaves chalk dust behind that can get on one's clothes. A good may be valuable in different ways at different times, depending on the context in which one values it. For example, the way a child values a piece of chalk in a classroom, as a means through which to learn a lesson, is different from the way the child values the chalk when wanting to play hopscotch.

Because goods are valuable for different reasons at different times, different people may concurrently value a good in different ways. I may value the piece of chalk as being a useful way to communicate my message to you, but you may value it because it reminds you of your youth. In these circumstances, we both can value the chalk in our separate ways. Situations arise, however, in which the ways two people value the same good conflict. If one person values a sexual relationship with another as being the foundation of a long-term relationship while the other values the relationship as providing short-term enjoyment, a conflict is likely to ensue. Since both relationships and enjoyment are authentic—it is rational, in our society, to value things in terms of these modes of evaluation—the determination of which way one ought to value the sexual relationship is not clear.

One could argue, in the face of this difficulty, that although goods appear to be valuable in different ways at different times, there exists a more fundamental way to value the good in which the conflict could be resolved. For example, if we regard long-term relationships and enjoyment as two faces of the same mode of valuation, say pleasure, we could determine which of the two participants in the sexual relationship most values the relationship in accordance with pleasure. Alternatively, even if no such fundamental mode of valuation exists, there may be some way of measuring or ranking the different modes of valuation applicable to the good and resolving any conflict according to which mode measures or ranks higher. That is, if we say that enjoyment is less important a value than creating long-term relationships, then it is more appropriate to value the sexual relationship in terms of its contribution to a long-term relationship than as leading to short-term enjoyment.

The problem with both of these arguments is that each of us makes decisions about goods directly in accordance with our own particular set of modes of valuation and do not, in fact, translate these modes of valuation into more fundamental modes or rank them on any fixed scale. We make decisions about goods and the way in which we value them on an ad hoc basis in the context of the particular ways in which we value goods—how I value this sexual relationship with this person at this time of my life, given my other commitments and aspirations—and not in accordance with some general principle such as whether enjoyment comes behind/in front of the creation of long-term relationships. Those who argue for more fundamental modes of valuation or for a scale on which to rank modes of valuation have to demonstrate why our intuition about the way we make decisions relating to value is wrong.

If we cannot identify a fundamental mode of valuation or a scale on which to rank modes of valuation, then either we must live with the fact that conflicts exist for which there is no unique resolution or we must each ignore how others, with different modes of valuation, value the goods we care about. Not only does the latter solution ignore the possibility that we may each value a good in accordance with several conflicting modes of valuation, but it falls afoul of one of the principles of Western ethical thought: that we ought to respect each other, including the decisions each of us makes about our individual lives.

The Body as a Good

The human body is a good because people authentically value the body in accordance with many different modes of valuation. Of all the tangible goods that exist in the world, the human body is arguably the one that we value most diversely and in ways that are highly personal to each of us. It is the means through which each of us experiences the external world and the means through which each of us recognizes each other. It is also inherently valuable as a source of our identities and, on some views, as a representation of God. Thus, for both instrumental (that is, as a means to reaching some goal) and inherent (because of what the body is in itself) reasons, we, in this society, value the body deeply and heterogeneously.

In addition to valuing the body as a whole, we also value its components, whether these be organs, blood, cells, or DNA. We do so from two distinct standpoints: for being inherently valuable in themselves and for being instrumentally valuable in aiding human health. Blood, for example, is both inherently valuable as a representation of life and instrumentally valuable as being an important ingredient in the manufacture of pharmaceutical and other health-preserving products.

While we do not necessarily value the body in exactly the same way as its components, we often value them in a similar fashion. We value both our bodies as a whole and our DNA, for example, as a representation of our uniqueness, we value the similarity between our bodies and between our blood as symbols of community, and we value the donation of the labor of our bodies and of an organ in terms of sharing. The differences that do exist between the modes of valuation that we apply to the body on the one hand, and to its components on the other, largely result from the strong link between the body's components and human health.

Human health, like the human body, is itself authentically valuable. Health is inherently valuable as a state of being in which we suffer neither pain nor illness. It is also instrumentally valuable as a state of being in which we can accomplish valuable tasks. Thus, to preserve one's health may be an obligation not only to oneself but to one's family and community. Alternatively, or in addition, we may impose on society the obligation to maintain its citizenry's health regardless of individual ability to pay.[11] The significance of health is further reflected in the rich metaphorical work to which we put it. We talk, for example, of sick or healthy economies and communities, of healthy attitudes, and of healthy servings of food.

There is one further significant difference between the ways in which we value the body and its components. Since components of the body may be altered through biotechnological processes, we must distinguish between valuing body components as they are on removal from the body and as they are after being transformed through biotechnology. This distinction between components in their unnatural—since the components are not generally found separate from the body in nature—but untransformed state and these components in their transformed state does not arise in relation to the body itself. This distinction between untransformed and transformed states is important since the transformation process may not only change the component itself but the ways in which we value it after transformation. Specifically, some of the ways in which we hold body components to be inherently valuable may not be applicable, or at least less significantly applicable, to the transformed component.

Consider, for example, the transformation of blood into plasma and into certain enzymes found within the blood. Blood itself is, in Judeo–Christian societies, a symbol of life; plasma and (to an even lesser extent) the extracted enzymes are less strongly associated with life. But while the transformation process leads to the diminution of some modes of valuation that were applicable to the untransformed body component—here, as a symbol of life—it leads to an increase in others, principally those relating to human health. That is, the primary way in which we value plasma and extracted enzymes is instrumentally in terms of their effect on increasing human health.

While the less transformed a body component is, the more it is valuable in the same way as the body and, conversely, the more transformed it is, the more it is valuable in the same way as human health, given the similar ways in which we value the human body and human health, the difference between the ways we value different goods falling within the definition of human biological materials is more one of emphasis than of kind. That is, while one would not likely value a transformed body component in exactly the same manner as one would value the body as a whole or an untransformed component, one would generally value it in a similar fashion.

A difference does arise, however, between untransformed body components and components that have been so transformed that they are no longer recognizable as a body component. This difference arises from our ignorance of the origins of the transformed component in that we no longer associate it with the body. This distinction thus has little to do with the way in which we would value the body component if we knew of its bodily origins and much to do with our ignorance of this origin. To the extent, however, that we disassociate the transformed component from the body, we have little reason to value that component as we do the body itself; we would likely, however, have much reason to continue valuing that component for its effect on human health.

It would appear that we ought not to have any concern that our application of property law to components that we have disassociated from the body will discourage modes of valuation that are peculiar to the body. In other words, even if property discourse, for example, discourages us from valuing goods in terms of identity, we may have no concern in applying this discourse to a body component that we have disassociated from the body even though we would be concerned in applying property discourse to the body itself. Although in some abstract sense a disassociated body component may be valuable in terms of identity—that is, if we knew that the component had been derived from the body, we would have valued it in terms of identity— it would seem that we need not concern ourselves with this mode of valuation in practice since we do not, in fact, value the component in terms of identity.

Before jumping to the conclusion that we may safely ignore those modes of valuation that we do not in fact adopt in relation to a disassociated body component, we should remember that what we are concerned about is not how we actually value particular goods but the manner in which we allocate rights of control over those goods. At the extreme, even if none of us value a disassociated body component in accordance with some mode of valuation, we may still be concerned about allocating that component on a basis that ignores that mode of valuation where that mode of valuation is important to the way we actually value the body. This is so because, at some point, the disassociated component was part of a living human body. If we are ready to allocate rights of control in the disassociated component without reference to mode of valuation X, then when faced with a decision about how to allocate rights to the precursors of that component, the force of precedent would militate in favor of us again allocating rights without reference to X. If we care about mode of valuation X, then as we move backward through the chain that led to the disassociated component, we risk allocating rights of control to goods that we value strongly in terms of mode of valuation X without reference to that mode of valuation. This is, admittedly, a thin edge of the wedge argument, but given that legal decisions are made on the basis of precedent and incremental change, it is nevertheless of real concern.

In reality, however, while the majority of the population may not associate a particular pharmaceutical as having been derived from the body, those who create pharmaceuticals very much have this knowledge. Since these are individuals who transform human biological materials into disassociated components, we ought still to care how these individuals value the component. Their decisions about what to do with these components strongly influences the nature of research conducted on the human body and relating to human health.

Property and the Body

Ultimately, this book is about how to allocate rights of control over human biological materials so as to do no injury to the ways that we, in this society, value the human body and human health. Since the principal means through which we allocate these rights is through the law of property, we must ask how treating something as the subject of property rights affects the ways in which we value the body and health. Those who practice property law do so against a backdrop of assumptions and conceptions, including many relating to reasons for and against allocating rights in certain goods. To the extent that these assumptions and conceptions favor allocating rights on the basis of the way individuals value the good in question or the way in which we value the individual to whom we grant rights, we give voice, in property discourse, to only a subset of all the possible ways to value the good.

*   *   *

In this book, I examine the likely effect on the ways in which we value the body and human health of subjecting the human body and health to property discourse. In chapter 2, I begin this examination through the analysis of one of the few judicial pronouncements directly on the question of who owns human biological materials. Through this analysis, I draw out three questions that I address in the remainder of this book. These are as follows. First, which modes of valuation do we encourage when we allocate rights of control through property discourse? Second, in which ways do we, in this society, value the human body and human health, and how do these ways differ from the modes of valuation encouraged through the application of property discourse? Third, given the differences between the way we value the body and health and the modes of valuation implicit within property discourse, can we nevertheless deal with the discouraged modes of valuation within property discourse?

My focus in chapters 3 through 6 is to investigate the first of these questions, that is, which modes of valuation do we encourage when we use property discourse? I undertake this investigation in four parts. In chapter 3, I set out the general thesis that, through property discourse, we allocate rights of control over a good so as to place the good, in some form, within the market. That is, we allocate rights of control to those individuals who value the good according to market modes of valuation. These modes of valuation include, for example, use value, ability to trade the good for another, and the ability to pass on the good on one's death. Call these modes of valuation *economic modes of valuation.*

In chapters 4 through 6, I examine the way that judges, who are the ultimate arbiters of legal discourse, decide whether to allocate rights of control over goods that have not, before those decisions, been the subject of property rights. In chapter 4, I study two goods, computer programs and nonhuman biological materials, in which, with one notable exception, those seeking rights of control had little or no interest in noneconomic modes of valuation. In chapter 5, I turn my attention to the human personality. Here, those seeking rights to this good valued it in accordance with both economic and noneconomic modes of valuation. Finally, in chapter 6, I analyze two cases in which the party seeking rights valued the sought-after good for primarily noneconomic reasons.

Through this examination, I illustrate that the courts, regardless of the actual basis on which individuals value a particular good, allocate rights to the good so as to encourage economic modes of valuation. That is, courts allocate rights of control to those individuals who present themselves to the court as valuing the contested good in terms of economic modes of valuation, whether or not these individual also value the good in noneconomic ways. The result is that, through property discourse, we encourage people to value goods that we call "property" in accordance with economic modes of valuation and discourage them from valuing these goods in noneconomic ways.

I turn next, in chapter 7, to answer the second question, in which ways do we value the human body and human health? My answer there expands upon the discussion in this chapter by examining some of the anthropological literature applicable to these goods. We have a complex understanding of our bodies and our health and have no less intricate ways of valuing both of these goods. Many of the ways we value our bodies and our health are contradictory in that should we act on one of the ways in which we value the body, we would undermine some of the other ways we value the body. Since many of these ways of valuing the body and health turn out to be noneconomic, there are large gaps between the modes of valuation we apply to the body and health and those implicit in property discourse.

To address the third question—whether, despite the differences between the ways we value bodies and health and the modes of valuation encouraged through the application of property discourse, can we nevertheless apply property discourse to human biological materials—I turn to the literature relating to the philosophy of value to determine whether, despite our focus on economic modes of valuation when engaging in property discourse, we are, through this discourse, nevertheless able to appropriately value the body and health in terms of all the ways that we, in fact, value them. In chapter 8, I examine whether we, through a discourse premised on encouraging economic value, are able to translate other, noneconomic, values into a money price and thus allocate rights of control through a ranking of these translated money prices. Since I conclude that this is not possible, principally because modes of valuation cannot be translated into each other, I discuss, in chapter 9, whether we can supplement property discourse with other discourses in order to consider all values. Given the nature of property rights, as providing the holder with a veto over the good subject to those rights, I argue that any supplementary discourse would likely be drowned out by property discourse.

My argument throughout this book is not that the human body or human health can never be appropriately valued in terms of economic modes of valuation; it is simply that economic modes of valuation do not exhaust the ways in which we value the body and health. The conclusion that I reach is not that we should not allocate rights of control over human biological materials, but, rather, that we must construct a method of allocating rights of control over these materials that take all modes of valuation, both economic and noneconomic, into account.

This book ends with the beginning of another by sketching out possible ways that we could create a scheme to address all modes of valuation inhering in human biological materials. While these sketches are described in broad strokes, my intention in putting them forward is to begin the debate about what form and shape these schemes ought to take. While perhaps no scheme will satisfactorily address all the modes of valuation applicable to human biological materials, I am confident that we can construct some method that would represent a significant improvement over property discourse.

2

Property Discourse and the Body

In an era when parts can be routinely detached from one body and plugged into another; when the U.S. National Institutes of Health offer to replace corpses in medical schools with 'industry-standard digital cadavers'; when certain machines can appropriate the functions of human organs, while others are invested with intelligence; when the life of the body can be prolonged when the mind has ceased to function; when genetic change can be engineered and human beings cloned; when a foetus can be nurtured in an artificial womb, or jobbed-out to a surrogate mother; when we entrust automatons to land our jets or perform operations on our bodies; when the *New York Times* informs us that, contrary to what most of us had believed, there are three, four or possibly five genders; when we capriciously rebuild faces, breasts or thighs to conform to the moment's ideal of beauty; and when we dream of 'Robocops', 'Terminators' and 'Replicants', and long to live in a *virtual* reality—then concepts and definitions, values and beliefs, rights and laws, must be radically overhauled. [1]

If all goes according to plan, scientists will have sequenced the entire human genome by the year 2005.[2] The goal of this sequencing effort is to furnish researchers and physicians with sufficient information that, using the tools of biotechnology, they will be able to combat disease and ailments through the synthesis of human hormones and enzymes, the development of new drugs, and, eventually, the use of gene therapy.[3] As this research effort leads to the development of new therapies, new pharmaceutical products, and new research tools, we can expect researchers and those who fund them to increasingly make claims to control these new therapies, products, and tools.

These claims have traditionally been stated in terms of property rights, specifically patent rights.

In this chapter I begin the analysis of whether we, as a society, ought to grant these researchers rights of control over human biological materials and, more generally, whether we ought to grant anybody such rights. Before embarking on an analysis of the advisability of applying property discourse to human biological materials, we need to determine whether there is anything peculiar about human biological materials that should cause us to hesitate before we allocate rights of control over these goods. There are two aspects of human biological materials that merit notice. First, as discussed in chapter 1, many of the products of biotechnological research on human biological materials are compounds commonly found in the human body or are components of the body itself. These products include, for example, insulin and other hormones, healthy and cancerous human cells, immunological agents, and DNA sequences that code for human proteins. Second, these products are most often used in curing or preventing human disease.[4] That is, the primary scientific interest in these compounds is their effect in promoting human health. For example, scientific discovery has allowed patients suffering from diabetes and similar hormonal diseases to self-administer insulin and other hormones; physicians treat cancer patients with various immunological agents;[5] and, should gene therapy become feasible, physicians will introduce DNA sequences into patients' cells in order to control genetic disease.[6]

Because human biological materials either are body components or derive from body components, their value to us is closely allied to the ways in which we value the human body. Given this nexus, the advent of modern biotechnology and the claims of the researchers who practice it will soon present us, for the first time since the abolition of slavery, with the necessity of deciding whether the human body and its components ought again to be the subject matter of property discourse. This is a task that we must undertake with care since, as discussed in chapter 1, the human body is a good that we value in many and contradictory ways.

In this chapter I open the debate about whether human biological materials ought to be considered as property by examining the setting in which this decision is likely to be made: in the courts. While Congress could, theoretically, make this determination itself, the legislative process is slow enough that those seeking rights of control over human biological materials will likely commence court actions well before Congress formulates any policy with respect to these materials. In addition, Congress may well wish to see how the courts determine the issue of ownership of human biological materials before acting.

As discussed in chapter 1, the allocation of rights of control over human biological materials through the application of property discourse gives rise to three distinct questions. The first of these questions is which modes of valuation do we encourage and which do we discourage through the application of property discourse? As discussed in chapter 1, we grant property rights in a good to an individual either because of the way that individual values that good or because of some characteristic of the individual. Either way, as argued in chapter 1, we allocate rights of control on the basis of a subset of all the ways one could value the good in question. Through my analysis of case law in this chapter and in chapters 3 through 6, I conclude that in awarding property rights, we value goods exclusively in accordance with economic modes of valuation, including market price, the ability to use, the ability to sell or transfer, the ability to inherit, and the ability to consume. This narrow focus to property discourse did not evolve through a lack of concern for noneconomic modes of valuation; rather, it evolved because of the assumption that all noneconomic values can be translated into a market price through the individual assignment of a price, which price will depend on how valuable, overall, that good is to the individual in question. The market will then allocate the good to that individual who values the good the most—as demonstrated by the price she or he is willing to pay for it—resulting in allocations that maximize overall value. In chapter 8, I examine the premises underlying this market analysis and find it wanting.

Second, how do the modes of valuation encouraged through the use of property discourse correspond to the ways that we value the human body, its components, and human health? I have already discussed some of the ways in which the human body and human health are valuable, but in chapter 7 I set these modes of valuation out in more detail. The discussion there illustrates the incredibly rich ways in which we value our bodies and our health, both as intrinsic goods and instrumentally to achieve other goods. My analysis ends with the conclusion that while property discourse is premised on economic modes of valuation, the ways in which we find the human body and human health to be valuable are principally, although not exclusively, noneconomic. Thus, there is little accord between the modes of valuation implicit in property discourse and the ways in which we hold the body and health to be valuable.

While the discord between the ways that we actually value the human body and the ways that, through property discourse, we value goods we call property may appear to be of academic interest only, the effect of this discord is very real. Should we allocate rights of control to those who value a good in terms of economic modes of valuation, we are necessarily not allocating those rights of control to those who value the good in noneconomic ways. Since those who have rights of control determine how the good will be used and for which purposes, the uses to which and the purposes for which those who value the good in economic ways would put the good will be favored at the expense of other uses and purposes. To the extent that those who value the good economically would use the good differently than would those who value it in noneconomic ways, the effect of allocating rights of control on an economic, rather than on a noneconomic, basis will be real and determinate.

The third question is, given that there is little correspondence between the ways in which we value the body and health and the modes of valuation encouraged through the application of property discourse, is it nevertheless appropriate to apply property discourse to human biological materials on the basis that property discourse can be modified to include other values, that these other values are translatable into modes of valuation encouraged by property discourse, or that we can supplement property discourses with other discourses that encourage noneconomic modes of valuation? I examine this question in chapters 8 and 9. I first conclude that it is not possible to translate one value into another or to translate all values onto a common scale on which they can be ranked. Second, I argue that while property discourse may be flexible in the long term, and thus may, in the future, come to encourage noneconomic values, anything that we call property will, in the short term, be allocated exclusively on the basis of economic values. Third, because property rights are both positive and negative, they trump other discourses. Therefore, it is very difficult to displace a property right, once granted, in order accommodate other discourses.

Interpreters of property law, should they treat the human body and human health as subject to property law and, thus, value them in accordance with economic modes of valuation, are likely not only to ignore the noneconomic aspects of these goods but also to resist addressing these noneconomic aspects when specifically raised. They will so resist because they believe that the market is the mechanism best equipped to deal with these aspects in a neutral manner. This belief is the source of much difficulty. The primary problem with it is that it prematurely arrests discussion in the courtroom about how best to promote all of the values inhering in a particular good. Judges and lawyers, wishing to appeal to neutral methods of choosing among competing claims, rely on the market to balance the plethora of ways of valuing a good. For example, by assuming that the market will assign a price to safety concerns, to the value of autonomy, to the value of self-development, and to the value of equality, courts and attorneys can claim that they are addressing all needs and wants while being relieved of the obligation of actively discussing and evaluating them. Since the market cannot sensibly assign a price to many values inhering in the human body and human biological materials, such values will be ignored in the formulation of judicial opinions concerning the body and such materials. Thus, by relying on the market, we risk making judicial decisions that fail to adequately balance the competing needs of members of our society with respect to these goods.

The Patient's Body

While there have been relatively few court decisions touching on the admixture of property law and the human body, one case, *Moore v. Regents of the University of California*,[7] provides a setting in which to discuss the effect of using property law to regulate biotechnological research in the human body. In 1976, John Moore sought treatment at the Medical Center of the University of California, Los Angeles, for hairy-cell leukemia, a rare disease. Dr. David Golde, the attending physician, confirmed the diagnosis and recommended that Moore's spleen be removed. Moore consented to the splenectomy, which was subsequently performed. On several occasions over the next seven years, at Golde's direction, Moore returned to the Medical Center.[8] During these visits, Golde withdrew samples of Moore's blood, skin, bone marrow, and sperm. Golde told Moore that these samples were required to monitor and ensure Moore's continued health.

During the period beginning with his first encounters with Moore, however, Golde recognized that Moore's body was overproducing certain important components of the human immune system, known as lymphokines. Golde perceived that the overproduction of the typically scarce substances made their isolation possible. Moore's cells, he realized, could be used as factories to produce lymphokines in large quantities, offering the opportunity for commercial exploitation.[9] In order to capitalize on this idea, Golde arranged before the splenectomy to have portions of Moore's spleen retained for research. Golde used the spleen tissue and the additional bodily substances collected from Moore during his subsequent visits to the medical center to create a culture of cells producing lymphokines. This cell line differed from Moore's ordinary cells only in that, through a well-known but sometimes difficult process,[10] the cells in the cell line were enabled to reproduce themselves indefinitely.

Realizing the enormous commercial potential of the cell line and its derived products—estimated to be approximately three billion dollars[11]—Golde and his research assistant, Shirley Quan, entered into contracts with several pharmaceutical companies and the University of California to commercially develop the cell line. Through these contracts, Golde received a substantial number of shares in one of the companies, and both Golde and the university were generously paid. Golde and Quan applied for and obtained a patent in the cell line and its derived products, which they transferred to the university.

Golde never informed Moore that the spleen and other cells were commercially valuable, nor that Golde intended to exploit this value for himself. When Moore discovered Golde's activity, he brought suit claiming that Golde, Quan, the university, and the pharmaceutical companies had taken—or, in legal terminology, converted—his cells and ought to disgorge the profit made from the cell line. Moore's claim was rejected on a preliminary motion at trial. On appeal, however, the California Court of Appeal found that Moore had retained a proprietary interest in his cells and that Moore was entitled to compensation for conversion if he could prove his claims at trial.[12] On further appeal, the Supreme Court of California found that Moore had no proprietary interest in his removed cells and thus could not sustain his action for conversion.[13] The court nevertheless held that Moore was entitled to compensation if he could prove that Golde had breached his fiduciary obligations to Moore by failing to inform Moore, prior to the splenectomy and the other medical procedures, of Golde's commercial interest in his cells.[14]

Two property claims were in conflict in *Moore*. While academic commentators have concentrated exclusively on Moore's claim to ownership of his spleen and other bodily cells,[15] the scope of Golde's property claim to these cells was also in issue. Golde's right to control the use of and profits from the human biological materials in question was clearly dependent on the extent to which the court recognized Moore's property interest in his removed cells. Given that the California Supreme Court declined to recognize the latter interest, Golde was left with plenary authority, within the bounds of health and safety regulations and patent law, to control and profit from the cells. Since the property interests of both Moore and Golde are fundamentally connected to one another, in analyzing *Moore*, it is wise to keep in mind both the nature of Moore's claim to his own bodily tissues and the nature of Golde's claim over the cells and related biological materials.

The *Moore* court spoke through four separate opinions, two for the majority and two in dissent. Each opinion reveals a different understanding of property law and of its application to the human body. These understandings emerge from the opinions indirectly, as the sum of each writer's bold strokes and small flourishes rather than through direct presentations. In this chapter, I examine what these different understandings reveal about the nature of property discourse and the likely impact of this discourse on the human body. I do this instead of enquiring into which of the four opinions best accords with current legal precedent not only because there is a plethora of commentary on the subject and, as this commentary amply reveals, there is no clear correct result, but because I am interested in discovering the nature of property discourse.

My first aim in investigating the *Moore* opinions is to explore the debate that unfolded therein over whether property discourse, as carried out in the courts, operates by valuing goods as commodities. One faction held that goods are only considered property when to do so facilitates the workings of the market. For example, goods such as friendship and sharing, which cannot be traded on a market without fundamentally altering the cultural meanings of each, are not property. On the other hand, pens and paper clips are property because they are capable, given current cultural understandings, of being traded on a market. Trade is enhanced when property rights are assigned in pens, but not when property rights are allocated in friendship. Thus, on this view, property rights attach to economic goods, goods that are traded or capable of being traded on the market. In contrast, the other faction argued that property rights attach to any good that is valuable, whether that value is a market price or some other concern such as autonomy or self-development. According to this view, courts assign property rights in order to further all values, not simply economic value. When a court determines that these values are best promoted by assigning a property right, it does so; otherwise, it refrains from granting such a right. Continuing with the earlier example, the value of mutuality is embodied in friendship in that, by its nature, friendship must be freely given and may be just as freely withdrawn. This value is best promoted by withholding a property right to a friendship since, if the courts were to recognize such a right, friendship, once given, would be compulsory and no longer voluntary.

My second aim in analyzing *Moore* is to examine whether, if there is in fact a nexus between property law and economic value, it is a wise policy to view human biological materials as property. Specifically, I examine the argument, expressed in one opinion, that the allocation of rights of control over and use of these materials solely on the basis of economic considerations compromises noneconomic values such as dignity and self-development. While later chapters will focus in greater depth on this issue, the *Moore* opinions illustrate the difficulty of protecting noneconomic values when property rights are allocated on the basis of market factors.

The Majority: Property as Enhancing Trade

The majority opinion in *Moore* belongs to the first faction described under my first aim; that is, the majority valued goods (here Moore's cells and tissues) in terms of their economic value. The majority's primary concern in dealing with Moore's conversion claim was the effect that a decision in favor of Moore would likely have on research and development in pharmaceutical products. Granting Moore a property right in his own tissues, the majority held, would impede future research and development using human biological materials. Every researcher into whose hands a patient's tissue passed would be liable

for conversion unless the patient had previously agreed to sell the tissue. Researchers would be unwilling to use tissues collected by others because of uncertainty over whether the donor of the tissue had adequately consented to the use of the tissue for research and commercial development. Such tissues would amount to "a ticket in a litigation lottery."[16] Similarly, "companies [would be] unlikely to invest heavily in developing, manufacturing, or marketing a product when uncertainty about clear title exists."[17] Therefore, the grant of a property right to Moore in his own tissues would hinder the free exchange of human biological materials and would, ultimately, lead to a reduction in the production of pharmaceutical products.[18] Since the allocation of a property right to Moore in his tissues would hinder trade in these tissues, the majority concluded that Moore ought not to be granted a property right. On the other hand, because trade is enhanced by granting researchers and pharmaceutical companies property rights to human biological materials, since this encourages heavy investment in the development and production of new drugs that will be traded on the market, property rights ought to be granted to such researchers and pharmaceutical companies.

Although the majority did not consider nonmarket values in its rejection of Moore's property claims, it did not ignore these values or treat them as insignificant; rather, the majority recognized that the human body is valuable in ways beyond its market price. In fact, in order to address the body's importance to individual autonomy, the majority extended the law of informed consent to require physicians such as Golde to inform their patients of any commercial interest they may have in their patients' tissues. By granting Moore the right to be informed of Golde's commercial interests, the majority sought to protect Moore's ability to make autonomous medical decisions.[19] When deliberating over whether to undergo the splenectomy, the majority held, Moore should have possessed information pertaining not only to the benefits and dangers of the operation itself but also to the quality of the advice Golde was providing to him. The majority sought to guarantee the latter type of information by requiring physicians to inform patients of factors, such as outside commercial interests, that a patient may reasonably believe to have influenced the physician's recommendations.

It is notable, however, that the majority was unwilling to go beyond its extension of the law of informed consent and invoke the law of property to protect Moore's autonomy.[20] This unwillingness prevailed despite the fact that the informed-consent remedy is less effective in reaching the goal of autonomy than would be a property right. A patient facing serious illness is unlikely to withhold consent to a necessary medical procedure simply because an attending physician discloses a commercial interest in the patient's tissues. The physician, not the patient, possesses the expert knowledge required to determine treatment.[21] The patient is, therefore, in no position either to second-guess the physician's recommendations or to determine the impact that the physician's commercial interests played on the formulation of these recommendations. Thus, the requirement that physicians inform patients of potentially conflicting interests provides little check on the influence that these interests play on physicians' recommendations and only minimally enhances patients' ability to make autonomous medical decisions. On the other hand, a property right in tissue could be formulated to reduce the likelihood that a physician would be influenced by his or her commercial interests in a patient's tissue. If patients retained property rights in their tissues following surgical removal, patients would retain the right to dispose of their tissues following the successful completion of their treatment. At this time, the patient would be in a significantly better position to evaluate whether to consent to the commercial use of his or her tissues. The patient's position would have improved both because the patient would be less dependent on the physician's ability to treat the patient's illness and because the patient would no longer be living under the cloud of his or her illness. Such a property right also works to reduce the influence that physicians' commercial interests have over their medical recommendations. Because a physician must bargain with a patient for commercial rights to tissue after the completion of medical treatment, the physician is less likely to be influenced by commercial considerations when formulating and recommending such treatment.

Justice Broussard: Human Biological Materials Already Property

Justice Broussard, in his dissent, accepted the majority's equation of property rights with the enhancement of trade in market goods. He argued that human biological materials are, for better or worse, market goods.[22] Physicians, researchers, and pharmaceutical companies exchange such materials, increasingly for a fee, and apply for and receive patents for such materials as they would for any market good. Given that human biological materials are already traded on the market, Justice Broussard held, there is no reason not to recognize the patient's economic interest in this material.[23]

He stated that a property right could be fashioned to allow patients such as Moore to participate in the economic value of their tissues without impeding research and development leading to new pharmaceutical products. He proposed that, where a physician fails to adequately inform a patient of the physician's commercial interest in the patient's tissue prior to the removal of that tissue, not only should the physician be held liable for failing to fully inform the patient under the law of informed consent, but the physician, lacking consent for the commercial use of the tissue, should also be held liable in conversion for any profit derived from this tissue.[24] Patients, under this proposal, have a property right in their tissues prior to their removal. Where a physician removes tissue surreptitiously, knowing of its commercial value, the physician must disgorge any profits made. Since, as Justice Broussard pointed out, it is only in the rare case that a physician knows beforehand that tissue can be commercially exploited, this proposal does not jeopardize continued research using human biological materials. Tissue that is currently in wide circulation is unlikely to have been removed with the knowledge that it was commercially valuable and thus researchers, Justice Broussard continued, can freely use human biological materials without fear of being sued. In addition, even if a pharmaceutical company finds that it has inadvertently profited from material gathered by a physician who had failed to disclose a known commercial interest in that material, damages are likely to be limited. Since the most economically valuable part of a pharmaceutical product is derived from the work of the researcher and is not inherent in the material itself, pharmaceutical companies will unlikely face large damage awards and thus will not be deterred from the development of new pharmaceutical products. In formulating the property right he would award to Moore, Justice Broussard thus strongly countered the majority's principal argument that granting Moore a property right in his own tissues would impede the future development and trade in pharmaceutical products.

The majority's contention that human biological materials are not property, Justice Broussard next argued, is simply false. Even though the majority did not recognize Moore's property interest in his own tissue, the majority recognized that Golde and the pharmaceutical companies possessed a property right to the biological material.[25] In effect, Justice Broussard wrote, the majority simply transferred Moore's property right to his tissue, including the right to profit therefrom, to Golde and the pharmaceutical companies:

> [T]he majority's holding simply bars *plaintiff*, the source of the cells, from obtaining the benefit of the cells' value, but permits *defendants*, who allegedly obtained the cells from plaintiff by improper means, to retain and exploit the full economic value of their ill-gotten gains free of their ordinary common law liability for conversion.[26]

While the market price of a patient's tissues may be a windfall to that patient, just as the market price of oil discovered on a piece of real property is a windfall to the landowner, Justice Broussard argued that this is no reason not to allow the patient to retain this price and is certainly no justification for rewarding those who misappropriate it.

The disagreement between the opinions of the majority and of Justice Broussard center on how best to promote trade in biological materials and in new pharmaceutical products. As already discussed, Justice Broussard carefully addressed the majority's concern that trade would be undermined if Moore were granted a property right in his own tissue by creating a narrow property right unlikely to stunt future research and development. While the majority obfuscated the question of whether human biological materials are property, Justice Broussard clearly accepted that, whether the courts like it or not, the pharmaceutical industry already treats such materials as market goods. The central question is, he reasoned, not whether human biological materials ought to be property but who should be permitted to control and profit from this property. There is no justification, he concluded, to exclude individuals such as Moore from participating in this extant market. To this the majority appears to have no answer.

The agreement between the majority and Justice Broussard is as significant, however, as their disagreement. Both analyze the question of whether the court ought to grant Moore a property right in his own tissue in terms of the effect such a decision is likely to have on the markets in human biological materials and pharmaceutical products. Both accept that functioning markets is the goal of their deliberations. Both agree that the effect their decision is likely to have on various factors such as the safety of biomedical research, the physician–patient relationship, and the self-development of individuals need not be explicitly addressed. The majority justified this position on the assumption that the market will neutrally sort out these factors. Underlying this assumption seems to be the belief that, to the extent that any explicit discussion of these factors is warranted, it should be undertaken as part of a larger discussion of the law of informed consent. Justice Broussard may not have believed that the market is fully up to the task of weighing all factors but he, nevertheless, accepted that it was not the court's role, in property-law decisions, to deal with such factors.[27]

The two remaining opinions in *Moore* diverge significantly from the points on which the majority and Justice Broussard agree. Fundamentally, both of these remaining opinions reject the premise that property rights in human biological materials ought to depend solely on the effect such rights are likely to have on the market. Both embrace the view that the human body and body tissues are valuable in ways beyond their market price and that such nonmarket values cannot be translated into a market price. Last, both agree that an appropriate analysis of the property law question in *Moore* must contend with these other values openly—that is, without assuming that the market will balance these values neutrally and invisibly.

Justice Mosk: Property as a Plurality of Values

Justice Mosk, in dissent, sought to bring all the divergent ways of valuing the human body and human biological materials within the scope of property law. He rejected the majority's and Justice Broussard's position that property discourse ought to be expressed in the language of the market. Specifically, he argued that courts ought not to grant or withhold property rights solely on the basis of market considerations; rather, they ought to ground their determinations on a host of values, many of which will have no market price.[28] Only by incorporating all values within its property analysis, Justice Mosk held, can the court hope to arrive at a decision that is both equitable and moral. In his discussion of the property law issue in *Moore*, therefore, Justice Mosk emphasized the need to recognize patients' inherent dignity and equalize the relationship between physician and patient.

Centrally, Justice Mosk contended that patients must be granted a property right in their own tissues if they are to maintain sufficient control over their bodies and themselves to accord with the requirements of human dignity. The majority's opinion, in narrowly focusing on market effects, failed, according to Justice Mosk, to address this most important of all values. While the economic arguments mustered by the majority are significant,[29] they ought not to have been controlling in the instant case. Nor can the majority take refuge by claiming that it considered nonmarket values in its informed-consent analysis. While Justice Mosk accepted this analysis as far as it went,[30] he challenged the majority's sterilization of property discourse from any infecting moral and ethical claims. He criticized the majority for its failure to investigate whether such claims could be better protected by a property right as opposed to a right of informed consent, and opined that the majority's decision to reject Moore's property right actually undermined the ethical and moral values inhering in the human body and human biological materials. While the former part of this assertion simply faults the majority for its lack of perception, the latter argument challenges the very basis upon which the majority proceeded.

Justice Mosk's challenge to the majority can be expanded. According to the majority, every value inhering in a good has a commensurate price in the market. Market forces invisibly tally these values and allocate the good so as to maximize overall value. By allowing the market to do its work, all values inhering in the good, such as dignity, self-development, and autonomy, are given their appropriate weight. Market allocations do not, therefore, endanger nonmarket values; they maximize them. This argument is premised on the belief that all values are commensurable, that there exists some scale of value on which every value inhering in a good can be placed and quantified. Through the process of commensuration, differences of nature or quality between specific values become differences in quantity of overall value. As discussed later, this contention is fundamentally flawed. The collapse of the distinction between the nature of a value—its particular pull on us, its interaction with our other values and with goals we have set for ourselves—and the quantity of overall value cannot be achieved without losing an appreciation of the intrinsic value of a good and of self-understanding.[31]

Assuming, for the moment, that values are not commensurable—that values cannot be placed on a single scale of value—one cannot be confident that the market will, as the majority hoped, consider and balance all of the various values inhering in human biological materials. Noneconomic values must be considered separately from market values, and decisions as to property rights ought to be made in light of an explicit balancing of all values. If the court only considers economic values in allocating property rights, then the court risks undermining noneconomic values that it has refused to explicitly consider. As suggested earlier, several noneconomic values are implicated in biotechnological research using human biological materials. These include respect for human bodies as the source of such materials, the safety of biotechnological research on the environment and on patients on whom the products of such research are used, and—because such products are directed to the provision of health care—the equitable and appropriate distribution of health care among the citizenry.

Of the identified nonmarket values implicated in the *Moore* case, the health care concerns in themselves demonstrate the difficulty of a property analysis based solely on market considerations. Such an analysis fails even if one accepts market discourse because market assumptions break down in the health care sector. The patient–physician relationship, for example, is unlike the arms-length commercial relationships upon which market norms are based. In this relationship, the patient not only "purchases" health care from the physician but entrusts the physician to select what ought to be purchased.[32] Thus the ideal of a rational, at least somewhat informed, agent is lost. Second, the cost of the selected health care is usually paid for by third-party insurers or the public purse.[33] The bargaining relationship between patient and physician, to the extent there is any, is limited more by the insurer's rules than by the direct monetary considerations of patient and physician. Third, the patient's health has strong effects on parties external to the patient–physician relationship, such as the patient's family, the patient's employer, and the patient's community.[34] These effects, being external to the market, are invisible to it. In sum, there is rampant market failure in the provision of health care.[35] Even assuming that all values are commensurable, this market failure casts serious doubt on the *Moore* majority's assumption that a strictly economic analysis of human biological materials can achieve a distribution of these materials that maximizes all values inhering in them.

The deficiency of a market analysis of health care and, with it, human biological materials is most apparent in its attempt to quantify, in terms of a market price, health status and pain. These aspects of health are hard to define[36] and notoriously difficult to quantify. For example, whether one measures a change in a person's health in terms of a fluctuation in that person's earning power, on the basis of that person's willingness to pay for an improvement in health, or in terms of a change in that person's life span, the technique chosen will be inadequate to the task. Valuing health in terms of earning power relegates the health of the elderly, the young, women, and racial minorities to a level below that of middle-aged white men, who are the highest income earners.[37] The willingness-to-pay approach is not only sensitive to wealth but provides vastly different results, depending on whether one measures individuals' willingness to pay before or during illness.[38] Measuring health in terms of years of life fails to account for the enjoyment of that life.[39] Two bedridden years in pain is hardly equal to two years of feeling fit, yet a market analysis based on life span would treat these as equivalent. The proposed remedy to this latter difficulty is to measure quality-adjusted life years;[40] but this solution simply brings us back to the question of how to measure the quality of a quality-adjusted life year.

Lurking behind any method of measuring health status is the larger obstacle of measuring pain and suffering. Because we can never truly anticipate pain's nature and impact on us, because we cannot clearly express this impact, and because we cannot rationally deliberate under the influence of severe pain,[41] any attempt to quantify the alleviation of pain in terms of price is impossible. Yet if pain cannot be measured nor the value of the alleviation of that pain be quantified, then neither can we appraise the value of improving a person's health status. The entire enterprise of measuring health on a scale of value is extremely precarious. Also hanging in this precarious position is the market price of human biological materials. After all, such materials derive much of their value directly from their ability to alleviate pain and increase health status. If the values of pain relief and health status cannot themselves be measured, then it is unrealistic to talk of a market price for such materials that in any way reflects the true values at stake.

A market analysis of human biological materials, based on the assumption that all values inhering in such materials can be assigned a market price, cannot live up to its underlying assumption. Justice Mosk pointed to two values, dignity and equity, for which the market is unable to provide a price. Other values such as the equitable distribution of health care, safety, and the community interest in the health status of all its members are similarly left out of the market's calculations. Unless, as Justice Mosk attempted to do, the court explicitly deliberates upon such values, the resulting property decision will fail to appropriately reflect all of the values inhering in human biological materials. A market analysis, such as the majority undertook, without a concomitant evaluation of nonmarket values leads, as Justice Mosk argued, to a result that "is both inequitable and immoral."[42]

Justice Arabian: Rejecting Property Discourse

Justice Arabian agreed with Justice Mosk that the court ought to openly address far more than market effects when deciding whether to grant Moore a property right in his own tissue.[43] He agreed that fundamental values were implicated in the *Moore* case:

> Plaintiff has asked us to recognize and enforce a right to sell one's body tissue *for profit*. He entreats us to regard the human vessel—the single most venerated and protected subject in any civilized society—as equal with the basest commercial commodity. He urges us to commingle the sacred with the profane. He asks much.[44]

Unlike Justice Mosk, however, Justice Arabian did not believe that these noneconomic values could be incorporated within a property-law analysis. He doubted both the institutional capacity of the court to discuss these values explicitly and the flexibility of property discourse to encompass these values. While Justice Arabian held that courts are institutionally incapable of balancing the myriad values involved in a case such as *Moore*,[45] his recognition of this lack of competence did not imply that the court ought to entrust the market to balance these values. Instead of a judicial or market solution to the problem of balancing values, Justice Arabian argued that the solution ought to be left to the legislature. Justice Arabian's approach contrasts strongly with the majority's view of judicial competence. The majority readily acknowledged that courts cannot explicitly weigh nonmarket values when allocating property rights; only the legislature is competent to do so.[46] However, to its mind, this was no reason to refrain from allocating property rights. Although courts cannot explicitly weigh nonmarket values in making their decisions, the majority suggested, courts can rely on the market to take such values into account by assigning each such value a price. Thus, the courts can do indirectly—and neutrally—what they could not do directly.[47]

Fundamentally, Justice Arabian believed that if the courts consider human biological materials to be property, the law would come to "treat human tissue as a fungible article of commerce," leading him to fear for "the effect on human dignity of a marketplace in human body parts."[48] Stated briefly, Justice Arabian did not want human biological products to become market goods. Treating these products as property, he feared, would subject them to a property analysis that treats all goods as market goods. In contradistinction to Justice Mosk, Justice Arabian did not believe that property discourse could encompass values beyond market values. Not only is the judiciary not competent to balance these values,[49] he contended, but the history of property discourse in the courts is premised on the belief that the market neutrally balances these values without the need for explicit consideration. This belief, which he did not accept, denies the need to expand property discourse to allow for an explicit discussion of nonmarket values. Until property discourse abandons its reliance on the market to maximize value, it will remain inhospitable to those arguing that property rights ought to be allocated on some basis other than the enhancement of trade. Doubting the market's ability to encompass all values and accepting that property discourse, as carried out in the courtroom, limits discussion to economic considerations, Justice Arabian forsook this discourse in order to protect nonmarket ways of valuing the human body. This was the only way to deal, he concluded, with a "question [that] implicates choices which not only reflect, but which ultimately define our essence."[50]

Justice Arabian's conclusion that market norms inherent in property discourse are incompatible with an open discussion and evaluation of nonmarket values carries with it a somber warning of the consequences of accepting the idea that human biological materials are property.[51] While property discourse falls into the difficulties described earlier, those engaged in the discourse remain unaware of these difficulties because of their assumption that the market encompasses and quantifies all values.[52] Therefore, without ever having consciously considered what is best for society, courts will establish a set of property rights and duties pertaining to human biological materials that promote certain values but not others. Moreover, which values are promoted and which are not will be more a function of chance than anything else. For example, granting researchers property rights in human biological materials and in the products of biotechnological research will likely skew research goals toward finding cures for disease and away from discovering the underlying social and environmental causes of disease. Because researchers and pharmaceutical companies profit from selling pharmaceutical products, they have no incentive to research how the lack of education, the lack of income, poor sanitation, and unsatisfactory working conditions cause disease, since such research is unlikely to result in profitable products.[53] In allocating to researchers and pharmaceutical companies property rights in human biological materials, the court would in effect be choosing a health policy that holds that health status is improved by access to better and newer treatments. Such a policy has, however, largely proved ineffective in improving health status.[54] In this hypothetical situation, the court would not arrive at this policy through deliberation on how best to improve the community's health status; rather, the court would arrive at this policy by its assumption that the market ensures that health status is maximized among the citizenry.[55]

Another example of an unconsidered policy choice produced through the allocation of property rights in human biological materials is the policy that disease ought to be viewed as an individual problem, specifically a problem of an individual's genetic code, instead of as a societal problem.[56] While this policy has been severely criticized,[57] the courts nevertheless encourage it by granting researchers and pharmaceutical companies property rights in human DNA and human proteins. Since such researchers and companies only profit if they can claim that their piece of DNA or their protein—instead of the environment, poor sanitation, or lack of adequate nutrition—is the cause of disease, they will conduct their research according to a model that understands disease to be located in an individual's genetic makeup.[58]

Even if, in the future, it turns out that health prevention becomes less effective than treating illnesses, or focusing attention on genetics becomes demonstrably superior to focusing on the physical and social environment in which we live, the fact remains that, through property discourse, courts will be allocating rights of control and thus skewing research goals and decisions, without engaging in any discussion concerning what would be the most appropriate health policy. In this book, I am not arguing for one health policy over another, but maintaining that the health policy we end up with ought to be the product of deliberation rather than of chance.

The disagreement between Justices Mosk and Arabian turned, at bottom, on Justice Arabian's rejection of the court's ability to expand property discourse beyond economic concerns. Justice Arabian believed that because human biological materials are so valuable in noneconomic ways, the court should not subject them to an analysis that would treat them as commodities. The values inhering in human biological materials, including the values inhering in good health, would be jeopardized in a discourse in which noneconomic values are assumed to be magically considered but are, in reality, ignored. Property discourse forecloses discussion of such policy concerns as the promotion of health status, the direction of future biotechnological research, and the nature of community through its false assumption that these policies will be appropriately and neutrally formulated through the market. Justice Arabian recognized that courts cannot replace their trust in the market with an explicit evaluation of values because the courts are institutionally incompetent to undertake such an undertaking. Accepting this lack of competency, he counseled the courts to exempt human biological products from property discourse and urged the legislature to intervene instead.

In this chapter I have begun to sketch out the principal areas of debate relating to the application of property discourse to human biological materials. The first of these involves the nature of property discourse and the effect this discourse has in guiding its participants to value goods we call property. Essentially, the question is whether, through property discourse, we allocate rights of control based on an examination of all values inhering in a good or whether we look only at economic modes of valuation in making these allocations. The second area of debate revolves around the ways in which we value the body, its components, and health, and whether the application of property discourse to these goods is likely to have a negative effect on the ways in which we value the body.

Justice Arabian claimed that property discourse, and the commodification that he feared it represented, did not permit a wide-ranging discussion on the values inhering in human biological materials; in fact, he worried that by submitting these materials to property discourse, we would lose some of the sanctity with which he valued the body. While Justice Mosk disagreed that we are limited by property discourse to economic modes of valuation, both he and Justice Arabian argued that human biological materials, the bodies they came from, and the health they promote are valuable in diverse ways that cannot be captured through economic modes of valuation alone.

The discussion in chapter 3 will focus on the area of disagreement between Justices Arabian and Mosk: the modes of valuation that are encouraged through the application of property discourse, specifically, whether property discourse encourages noneconomic modes of valuation such as community, respect, and sharing. In that chapter, which leads to detailed case analysis in chapters 4 through 6, I argue that Justice Arabian's view of property discourse—that it encourages only economic modes of valuation—most accords with the way legal practitioners apply property discourse. I present specific examples, in chapters 4 through 6, of courts rejecting property arguments based on noneconomic modes of valuation in support of this conclusion.

Chapter 7 returns to the area of agreement between the two judges, showing that there is a large variety of values inhering in human biological materials. In that chapter, I provide but a sample of the large body of support for the judges' intuitions concerning the diversity of values inhering in human biological materials.

Based on my conclusions with respect to issues both separating and uniting the opinions of Justices Arabian and Mosk, I claim that Justice Arabian correctly held it inappropriate to award property rights to patients such as Moore in the human biological materials retrieved from their bodies, because to hold otherwise would impose a discourse based on economic modes of valuation on goods that are valuable in largely noneconomic ways. Even his decision is, however, wanting since his conclusion not to award property rights to patients does not reverse the fact that researchers, such as Golde, continue to possess and exercise rights of control over those same human biological materials.

In chapters 8 and 9, I ask whether we ought to abandon property discourse in its entirety in relation to human biological materials or whether we can salvage our reliance on this discourse by finding ways to translate noneconomic modes of valuation into economic modes of valuation, by expanding the scope of property discourse, or by supplementing property discourse with other discourses. I conclude that values cannot be translated into other values or onto a common scale of value without doing serious harm to what we mean by those values and how we act upon those values. Second, while in the long term, property discourse may expand to include a direct consideration of noneconomic modes of valuation, given the nature of the law and legal reasoning, it is unrealistic to expect such a change in the near future. Third, since property rights are not only negative—that is, the right to prevent someone else from doing something—but positive—the right to direct the use and consumption of a good—there is little room for other discourses to allocate rights of control over human biological materials in such a manner as to encourage those modes of valuation left out when we participate in property discourse.

If we cannot reform property discourse to include other values and we cannot supplement property discourse through the practice of other discourses, then, given that human biological materials have not yet been fully subjected to property discourse, we should find some alternative means of allocating rights of control over these materials. In chapter 9, I sketch out what some of these schemes may look like.

3

Property Discourse Evaluated

No one is fully contented with his present fortune; all are
perpetually striving, in a thousand ways, to improve it. Consider any one of them at any period of his life and he will
be found engaged with some new project for the purpose of
increasing what he has. Do not talk to him of the interests and
the rights of mankind; this small domestic concern absorbs
for the time all his thoughts and inclines him to defer political
agitations to some other season.[1]

The Human Genome Project, the international effort to map the entire
human genetic sequence,[2] is, by all accounts, on track and is attracting
much attention from private financiers.[3] Venture capitalists are investing heavily in start-up companies to exploit the commercial potential of both the equipment and technology that will be used to sequence
the genome and the new human diagnostic and therapeutic products
developed as a result of the sequencing effort itself.[4] This investment
is significant not only in dollar amount,[5] but because these venture
capitalists are directing their money to companies the major assets
of which are their links to researchers conducting basic research in
biology.[6]

   The new interest of private investors in biotechnology and, more
fundamentally, the new collaboration between basic researchers and
venture capitalists signals a profound change in the way researchers
are likely to advance their science.[7] Top biologists, whose only conflicts
of interest, up to now, stemmed from their intellectual commitments,
now hold significant financial stakes in the outcome of their own and
their colleagues' work. This financial interest engenders new and
potentially large conflicts of interest for these scientists, from their
ability to peer review work in their field,[8] through their ability to
impartially assess raw data, to their choice of research goal.[9]

Intellectual property rights will likely be at the heart of the new conflicts of interest. This will be so because the links between researchers and biotechnology companies will be forged out of these rights. Researchers have and will continue to exchange the future products of their work for present funding of their research and a share in future profits.[10] The lure of commercial reward will increasingly lead scientists to create intellectual property, to protect this property from competitors, and to market the products of this property to physicians and patients. To what extent traditional research norms—the slow but methodical collection of data, the prompt and wide dissemination of findings, and the sharing of insights—will be displaced by commercial norms—finely targeted research, secrecy, and protection of ideas[11]—will in large measure depend on the nature of intellectual property rights and how they are protected.[12]

Moreover, any alteration in traditional research norms is likely to have effects beyond the laboratory. Specifically, should researchers target their work toward the discovery of genetic flaws, for which companies can develop therapeutic products, and away from the investigation of social and environment causes of disease, for which only social remedies exist, certain social changes may follow. Some authors have speculated that one such change may be a concomitant shift away from societal responsibility for disease and toward individual responsibility for illness.[13] As researchers concentrate their efforts on discovering what causes a particular individual to contract a certain disease—be it the individual's genome or the individual's lifestyle—little will be learned about social causes of disease—for example, pollution, the lack of adequate sex education, and uncertainty over future employment prospects. In addition, societal institutions such as schools and courts will come to rely on the tests and diagnoses provided by health care researchers: tests and diagnoses derived from a paradigm of individual responsibility for disease.[14] Therefore, while such tests and treatments promise an objective way to treat illness, they carry with them the assumption that disease is an individual problem and not a social one.

In the development and implementation of health and biotechnology policies, governments will have to contend with the effects that intellectual property rights in human biological materials are likely to have on research norms and the goals of biomedical research. Intellectual property rights, like all property rights, further certain, but not necessarily all, ways of valuing these materials. In order to assess the effect of these rights on health and biotechnology policies, we must determine what these ways of valuing are and how they relate to biotechnology and health care.

To call a good "property" is to subject it to property discourse. Property discourse is that combination of conceptions, assumptions, and language used by legal practitioners—judges, attorneys, and legislators—to decide to whom and in what circumstances we ought to grant rights of control over a good. In this chapter I will expand upon the discussion in the previous two chapters on the contents of property discourse and the modes of valuation that it encourages and discourages.

Human biological materials are now sufficiently valuable, in terms of profits and future research, to researchers and investors alike that one can expect both of these groups to claim rights of control over human biological materials. As these claims collide with the claims of those who value these materials for other reasons, as in *Moore*, we can expect more disputes to be brought to the courts for resolution. Before these claims reach the courts, and before Congress intervenes with its own solution, we have an opportunity to examine whether property discourse, the discourse that both the courts and Congress employ in resolving property law disputes, provides an appropriate way in which to discuss human biological materials and the values inhering in them. In particular, we must ascertain which modes of valuing human biological materials courts and Congress encourage through their decisions dealing with rights of control over these materials.

Property discourse has been created largely through past court decisions. Whenever individuals claim the right to use, to profit from, or keep a good, or the right to prevent others from doing so, they will voice their claim through legal practitioners and ultimately through a court action. While Congress may, at any point, legislate who ought to have which rights of control at which time, most decisions concerning the allocation and meaning of property rights are, in fact, resolved through the court system or by attorneys based upon their expectation of what the courts will say with respect to a particular dispute. It is therefore to the courts and to those arguing before them that we must look in order to investigate property discourse.

The investigation unfolding in this and the next several chapters will illustrate that courts find a good to be "valuable," and thus worthy of protection as property, when its dominant value to the parties is economic. Where a party can demonstrate that a good is economically valuable to that party—that the party will trade in that good on an open market—courts are likely to award property rights if to do so will enhance such trade. If, however, the parties cannot persuade a court that they value the good principally in terms of its economic value or the court perceives that the allocation of property rights to one or the other of the parties will, in fact, hinder trade in the good, the court is unlikely to award a property right. For example, in *Moore v. Regents of the Univ. of Cal.*,[15] discussed in the previous chapter, the parties successfully convinced the majority that their only interest in Moore's tissues was economic. The majority was thus willing to consider whether Moore ought to be granted a property right in his tissue. The majority rejected Moore's claim, however, because it believed that the award of a property right to Moore would stifle research using human biological materials. The majority arrived at this conclusion through its supposition that pharmaceutical companies would be unwilling to invest in research where the ownership of the results of this research was uncertain. Granting patients property rights in their tissue, the majority held, would create just such uncertainty. Because pharmaceutical companies would be unwilling to invest in biotechnology research and development—thus severely reducing the supply of new pharmaceutical products—the market in pharmaceutical products would be seriously compromised. As Justice Broussard noted, however, while the majority rejected Moore's claim, it was not adverse to recognizing that property rights exist in human biological materials. The majority opinion, he stated, recognized that researchers and pharmaceutical companies hold such rights in human biological materials; the only parties prevented from holding these rights were the patients from whom the tissues were extracted. The majority thus concluded that human biological materials belong to the class of goods to which property rights can attach—goods valued for their market price—but that, in the interests of furthering a market in these and related goods, these rights ought to be withheld from Moore.

Property's Inner Heart: Market Values

The academic literature affords little insight as to which modes of valuing goods courts seek to promote in allocating property rights. The received learning, extracted from this literature, is that the label "property" is best understood as the legal conclusion that a good is, in some way, valuable.[16] In what respect, however, the good must be valuable, and thus be worthy of protection as property, is unclear. A good, after all, can be valuable in myriad ways including its aesthetic attributes, its ability to provoke intellectual insight, its provision of comfort, its inspirational qualities, and its market price. For example, a building may be valuable in terms of the beauty of its architecture, the shelter it provides to its inhabitants, its quiet serenity that inspires creative contemplation, its history, and its price on the open market. The received learning fails to define which, if any, of these ways of valuing a good, either singly or in combination, motivates courts to label a good as property.

In this and the next three chapters, I examine case law rather than academic literature, since one of my goals is to discover the bases upon which property rights are currently being awarded and balanced rather than to determine on which bases property rights ought to be allocated. While the academic literature is rife with suggestions as to how property ought to be conceived, I am interested in revealing the conception of property that applies today to goods labeled "property." My ultimate goal in this book is to determine what is likely to occur if we, as a society, agree to consider human biological materials as property. Specifically, my goal is to determine whether property law is capable of adequately balancing the many values—including self-development, autonomy, and community, among others—that inhere in the human body. If property law is not capable of balancing these values, then, as I suggest in chapters 7 through 9, the human body and human biological materials ought not be subject to property rights.[17]

Since my goal is to map out the current conception of property as expressed in American courtrooms, I am not concerned with whether a specific case was properly decided. In the following chapters, I undertake to probe the opinions given in various property cases to discover the conception held by the judge or judges writing those opinions. Thus, my goal is not to criticize particular opinions; instead, I take a critical look at those opinions to discover the conceptual framework of their authors. In pointing out and challenging assumptions found in these opinions, my intent is not to demonstrate that the judges ought to have done something different or better; rather, I am parsing them to discover which assumptions are fundamental to the current conception of property and which are not.

Despite the coupling of property law analysis with a good's

market value as exemplified by *Moore,* courts appreciate that people value goods in ways other than the good's market price. Courts assume, however, that the price of a good on the market reflects all these modes of valuation. That is, courts believe that a good's market price is epiphenomenal of all the various ways in which people value that good. In the market, people attach a monetary price to the way in which they individually value a good. This monetary price is a function of many factors including, for example, whether possession of the good is essential to the way in which the individual values the good and whether the individual values other goods more than the good in question.

Consider, for example, several of the possible ways of valuing a wedding ring.[18] The jeweler who created the ring is proud of her skill as exemplified in the design and execution of the ring. The jewelery store manager values the ring as a means to derive an income on which to live. The wearer of the wedding ring values it, at least in the ideal case, as a symbol of mutual love. The jeweler, the manager, and the wearer, although valuing the ring in diverse ways, each will be willing to pay some price for it. The price each individual is willing to pay will be a function of how each values the ring. The manager, who views the ring as merely a means to achieve an income, will attach a lower price to the ring than would the jeweler, who views the ring as a unique expression of her creativity. The jeweler, in turn, will attach a lower price to the ring than the wearer, since possession of the ring is essential to the way in which the wearer values the ring—as a constant reminder of mutual love—but is not essential to the jeweler's mode of valuation—as a source of pride—since the jeweler can be proud of the ring from afar.[19] Since the wearer will be willing to pay the most for the ring on the market, the wearer will come to own it. Through this process of individual assessment of willingness to pay, the market ensures that the ring is put to its highest use:[20] as a reminder of mutual love. No other use of the ring will result in as much overall well-being as this use. If, for example, given the stated motivations of each of the parties, the jeweler were to repossess the ring, the slight increase in the jeweler's well-being brought about by having possession of the ring would not compensate for the wearer's distress in losing this unique symbol of mutual love.

The market, as thus described, offers courts the opportunity to ensure that goods are put to their highest use and to do so without having to make explicit value choices. The market provides a mechanism through which individual assessments of value, as translated into money prices, are objectively compared. This comparison is merely mechanical and involves no *a priori* determination of which modes of valuation ought to prevail. In relying on the market to find a good's highest use, therefore, courts can remain neutral as to how society ought to value the good. Given this understanding of the market, the courts confidently put aside any explicit evaluation of worth, trusting the market to rank the ways in which the good is valued. This has two benefits from the court's point of view. First, since courts refrain from making difficult policy decisions—the ranking of modes of valuation—they remain well within the boundaries of their institutional role: that of impartial arbiters. They thus avoid any question of institutional competency. Second, the market provides the courts with a relatively straightforward method of allocating property rights. Courts do not have to struggle with and evaluate a large variety of frequently conflicting modes of valuation; they need only examine goods from one standpoint: the economic one. Parties who cannot explain in economic terms why the court ought to grant a property right will not be granted such rights. Parties who cannot found their opposition to the grant of a property right on market principles will fail to block the allocation of property rights.

Later chapters will examine the premises upon which courts rely in trusting the market to sort out conflicting claims of value. Chief among these is the assumption that the amount of money an individual is willing to pay for a good is an accurate and complete reflection of the way in which that individual values the good. This premise is complicated by the fact that individuals often value a good in several ways simultaneously. The amount an individual is willing to pay for a good must, therefore, accurately reflect all the ways in which that individual values the good. This entails that each individual rank her or his ways of valuing a particular good and attach a price to the good in accordance with that individual's highest ranking mode of valuation. Only if it is true both that individuals can meaningfully rank the ways in which they value a good and that each individual's assessment of value can be accurately translated into a market price is the courts' reliance on the market to arbitrate between conflicting values justified.

Enhancing Trade through Property

This and the next three chapters examine property-law decisions issued by state and federal courts, with special emphasis on those dealing with intellectual property claims (such as, for example, patents and copyright) in order to determine which values courts deem relevant to their decision whether a good is to become the subject of a property right. This chapter begins the discussion by positing the thesis that the only values courts directly consider in their determination of whether a good is property are economic values. Specifically, courts award property rights in a good where the parties value the good primarily for its market price and where the existence of property rights encourages trade in that good. The next three chapters expand upon this thesis by examining cases in which, increasingly, the parties come to value the disputed goods in ways beyond their market price. The next chapter applies the thesis to inventions. This is followed, in chapter 5, by an examination of the courts' treatment of property claims in one's personality. Chapter 6 concludes the discussion by focusing on two cases in which the parties valued the disputed goods in primarily noneconomic ways: in one case in terms of artistic integrity and in the other in terms of community.

Two lines of discourse in property-law analysis point to the significance of market values in this analysis. These lines are frequently presented to courts ruling upon property claims to novel goods such as the cell line in *Moore v. Regents of the Univ. of Cal.*[21] The first of these lines is the argument that the grant of property rights in a good increases the stock of that good in society by rewarding those who produce it.[22] Thus, some critics of the *Moore* decision contend that the court ought to have recognized patients' property rights to their own tissue in order to increase the stock of desperately needed organs and tissues.[23] Those advancing the second line emphasize that the grant of property rights to new creations stifles further discovery and invention by limiting access to new ideas and by establishing monopolies over the use of these creations. This was essentially the argument put forward by the majority in *Moore* when it held that patients ought not to be granted property rights in their own tissue.[24]

These two lines of discourse, that property rights increase the stock of goods by rewarding invention and that property rights decrease the stock of goods by creating monopolies, are often heard together in property-law discourse. Congress and the courts, in designing and implementing patent law,[25] for example, consciously attempted to maximize creative activity by seeking the optimal balance between property rights and the free use of ideas and information.[26] To achieve this balance, the law at once provides inventors with the right to "make, use, or sell" the patented good but limits this right to a period of years and to the exact specification of the invented good. At the expiration of the patent right, the inventor's monopoly disappears. Members of the public are then entitled to use the invented good in any fashion they desire. By rewarding inventors, but not so much as to establish stifling monopolies, those who posit patent law rely on the market to maximize the creation and output of new goods.

Two cases, *Stanley v. Columbia Broadcasting System, Inc.*[27] and *Murray v. National Broadcasting Co.*,[28] dealing with the creation of a radio and television program idea, respectively, illustrate the judicial reliance on the market to increase the production of goods. Stanley developed the idea, script, and format for a radio program entitled "Hollywood Preview," in which plots for potential Hollywood movies would be previewed to the listening audience. The audience would then be asked to write in and comment on the plot and to suggest actors to play the various roles. If the plot found favor with the audience, it would be made into a movie. Prizes would be awarded to audience members who wrote the best letters. Stanley presented the idea, title, script, and format to officials at CBS on the understanding that he would be reasonably compensated should CBS decide to use the idea. Some time later, CBS began broadcasts of a new show with a title similar to that proposed by Stanley that previewed Hollywood movies that were in the process of being filmed. The studio audience, rather than the home audience, was asked to respond to the plot. Although at first no prizes were awarded, CBS began awarding prizes in later broadcasts of the program. Because of the similarity between his proposed program and that actually broadcast by CBS, Stanley commenced an action to recover damages for the misappropriation of his program idea. A jury found that the two programs were substantially similar and awarded Stanley $35,000. This verdict was upheld by the Supreme Court of California.

The principal issue before the supreme court was whether Stanley was entitled to a common-law copyright—the right not to have his idea copied—in his program idea and format. Given the jury's determination that Stanley's idea and the program eventually broadcast by CBS were substantially similar, if Stanley held such a copyright,

CBS would be liable for infringement of it. A majority of the court held that Stanley did indeed hold such a copyright. The majority reasoned that Stanley was entitled to copyright protection because his idea was new and novel. The novelty, the majority explained, was not in the creation of a new title, format, or the idea of audience participation but in the combination of these elements.[29] This combination, the majority held, ought to be rewarded because it represented "a real improvement" upon existing program ideas and "entailed the exercise of skill, discretion and creative effort."

The majority did not explain why individuals ought to be rewarded with property rights for having exercised skill, discretion, or creative effort. In fact, not all individuals who exercise skill, discretion, or effort are rewarded with rights. Philosophers who develop new understandings of human rights, physicists who discover new subatomic particles, entrepreneurs who develop new markets, and artists who found new aesthetic movements receive no such rights. Given this, the majority could not have been arguing that all creative efforts ought to be rewarded with property rights. While the majority did not explicitly state which creative efforts ought to be rewarded and why Stanley's efforts fell within this class, they did provide some clues.

One explanation—that will be drawn out in the pages to follow— for the majority's willingness to reward Stanley's creative efforts is that Stanley's idea was valuable in an important way: it had a market value. Ideas such as Stanley's were commonly traded between creators and radio broadcasters.[30] The majority's willingness to award property rights to Stanley stemmed from their desire to protect his idea's economic value rather than any other quality it may have had. The majority looked exclusively at economic considerations, ignoring other ways to value Stanley's idea such as its entertainment value, its educational value, its aesthetic value, or its value to Stanley as a source of pride.[31] Thus, the only relevant value for the purposes of property law, according to the majority's analysis, is a good's market price.

Justice Traynor, in dissent, argued that property rights ought to be allocated in such a manner as to foster creative effort.[32] He recognized that such effort was best promoted by granting property rights to the those engaged in certain forms of creative activity, but not in others. The development of new creations depended, he argued, upon the free flow of abstract ideas; he held, therefore, that such ideas should not be the subject of property rights.[33] On the other hand, creative effort was encouraged, in his view, by granting property rights to those who took these abstract ideas and, through skill and industry, transformed them into "concrete forms, uniquely their own." Justice Traynor thus found that the purpose of property law in this context is not to reward those who have expended skill and effort to create new ideas; otherwise he would have recognized the rights of philosophers and physicists in their discoveries. Rather, the goal of property law, Justice Traynor concluded, is "[t]o insure free trade in ideas" in order to maximize creative activity.[34]

According to Justice Traynor, the individual elements of Stanley's program idea lacked novelty.[35] He accepted, however, that even though the elements of an idea were "hackneyed," the combination of those elements could still prove sufficiently creative as to be novel. Such a fresh combination would be novel, Justice Traynor held, even if commonplace and dull, provided it was marketable, if it had "enough promise of winning the attention of the public." Stanley's idea was, however, merely "a fresh application of an idea that has thrived on repetition." As such, the program idea was more valuable because of its similarity to existing programs than because of any new twist on these programs. Justice Traynor held that Stanley ought not to be granted a property right in an idea that was marketable only because it was copied from familiar program formats.[36]

Of all the values inhering in radio programming—entertainment, aesthetic, educational, community, economic, etc.—Justice Traynor looked only to a program's market value.[37] Consider, for example, Justice Traynor's willingness to allocate property rights in the concrete formulations of abstract ideas but not in the abstract ideas themselves. Such an allocation of rights results in the maximization not of the quality, usefulness, morality, or aesthetics of inventions, but of their sheer number. Here Justice Traynor's reliance on the market comes back into play. Presumably, Justice Traynor was not oblivious to the quality or morality of inventions, even if he did not discuss these characteristics. By assuming, however, that the market would sort through all inventions and would attach the highest price to those that were of the highest quality, highest use, or highest morality, he was relieved of the obligation of discussing these characteristics explicitly. All property law had to do was to maximize the number of inventions. The market could then be trusted to pick out which of these inventions was valuable and reward these with a high price. Thus, through the combined work of property law and the market, society would become the beneficiary of the maximum number of valuable inventions. Overall happiness was thus guaranteed.

Murray v. National Broadcasting Co.[38] also suggests a link between property law and market value. In 1980, Murray submitted five written proposals to NBC for program ideas. One of these, "Father's Day," was a half-hour television show starring Bill Cosby as the devoted father of a closely knit African-American family. The show was to depict a compassionate, proud authority figure, in contrast to most depictions of black men on television. An NBC official asked Murray to expand on the "Father's Day" proposal and submit it to the NBC vice-president in charge of entertainment. Murray did so in a two-page memorandum in late 1980. NBC decided, however, not to pursue the idea and returned the memorandum to Murray soon after.

In the fall of 1984, NBC brought out a new series, "The Cosby Show." It starred Bill Cosby as the devoted father of a closely knit African-American family. This show soared in the ratings during its first season and became one of the most popular programs in television history. Murray commenced an action against NBC for the misappropriation of his idea. NBC maintained, however, that the idea for "The Cosby Show" had been developed independently of Murray.

A majority of the Court of Appeals for the Second Circuit found against Murray. Applying New York state law, they held that an idea must be "original or novel in order for it to be protected as property." Like the majority in *Stanley*, the *Murray* majority held that genuinely novel ideas ought to be protected through property rights; everything else ought to remain in the public domain.[39] Like the majority in *Stanley*, the *Murray* majority failed to explicitly state why these ideas ought to be so protected. Again, the answer may have been that genuinely novel ideas are generally marketable. The majority held that Murray's idea of combining a situation comedy format with the positive representation of a black family, while a breakthrough in the sense that no one had actually produced such a show, was not novel since many people, including Bill Cosby as early as 1965, had suggested just such a combination.[40]

Justice Pratt, dissenting, disagreed with what he considered the majority's overly strict definition of novelty.[41] In doing so, he established a link between the meaning of novelty and the market in program ideas. He held that in this market it was impossible to formulate a concept that had never before been expressed. Novelty, he continued, is subjective and varies over time as the market in programming changes. For Justice Pratt, then, the purpose of property law is not so much to reward invention for its own sake; rather, its purpose is to foster the development of marketable ideas. Justice Pratt, more clearly than the majority or either side in *Stanley,* stated which value inhering in inventions was relevant to property law: economic value.

The *Stanley* and *Murray* opinions, although separated by almost forty years, are similar in significant ways. The majority in *Stanley* and the dissent in *Murray* both argued that the law ought to reward certain creative efforts: those for which there is an extant market. The dissent in *Stanley* and the majority in *Murray* argued that only truly novel ideas ought to be treated as property. All four opinion writers shared a commitment to increasing the number of inventions. Behind this commitment lay the assumption that the market would ensure that only the most valuable—in terms of entertainment, education, etc.—of these inventions would survive. Since the market would ensure that overall value is maximized, courts need not explicitly consider values other than market values.

International News Service v. Associated Press: Economics at the Fore

To further illustrate that the courts rely on the market to sort out values and to expand upon the relationship between property law and the market in general, I turn next to the United States Supreme Court decision in *International News Service v. Associated Press.*[42] Starting with this case, I sketch out the two hurdles courts erect before agreeing to recognize a property right in a good. As stated earlier, the first of these is the requirement that the parties value the contested good primarily in terms of market price. Second, the party seeking the property right must satisfy the court that the grant of such a right furthers, rather than hinders, a market in that good.

International News Service arose during the First World War when certain foreign governments prevented the International News Service from collecting news on and sending news from their soil. In order to provide its member newspapers, numbering approximately 400, with war news, INS copied news stories from east coast member papers of the Associated Press. INS transmitted these stories, sometimes in identical form, to its west coast member papers which, because of the time difference between the two coasts, published the stories at the same time as west coast AP newspapers. Since INS and AP were competitors, AP took umbrage at what it considered the wholesale misappropriation of its news articles. AP brought suit, alleging that INS had engaged in unfair competition, and sought an order enjoining INS from continuing with its practice. A majority of the Supreme Court granted the order.

AP had little difficulty convincing the Court that both news agencies valued news in terms of market price. News services, AP argued, are in the business of collecting and distributing news. News stories are, therefore, the products from which news agencies profit.[43] The value of news, AP contended, is demonstrated by the fact that people are willing to pay for it. The "sole elements of value" inhering in news, AP continued, "are its novelty, its accuracy and its presence in the place where there are people interested enough to pay for knowing it, and at the time when they are so interested." In sum, AP argued that news was only valuable, from its perspective, as a commodity. AP did not value news as, for example, a means to support the war effort, as a way of helping families keep track of the fate of their loved ones, or as a means of developing a sense of community. For INS as well, news only had value as a commodity.[44]

The majority of the Supreme Court endorsed the view that the primary value of news is its market price.[45] The majority recognized that both INS and AP were in the business of collecting and distributing news; that news, from the perspective of the news agencies, was a commodity from which they could extract a profit.[46] The majority held, therefore, that the value of news depended on spreading it while fresh and that this value was lost once the news ceased to be secret. By holding, for the purposes of resolving the dispute between INS and AP, that news was valuable only while being held secret, the majority eschewed many other ways of valuing the news. If, for example, the majority had valued news in terms of strengthening the community then its value would have been enhanced, not lost, by sharing it with all members of the community. Similarly, if the majority had valued news in terms of its ability to inform families of the fate of their loved ones caught in the war, the value of news would have been greater when shared rather than when kept secret. Instead of valuing news along these lines, the majority directly equated the value of news with the price of news in the market. The majority thus stressed that news had an "exchange value" both to those who collect it and to those who would misappropriate it, that news was "saleable by [the] complainant for money," and that, to maintain the value of news, it was "essential that the news be transmitted to members or subscribers as early or earlier than similar information can be furnished to competing newspapers by other news services."[47]

For all this, the majority was reluctant to fully concede that AP had overcome the first hurdle to gaining a property right—that the only interests involved in the contested good were economic. This reluctance stemmed from the majority's recognition that newspaper readers, the general public, do not value news in terms of its market price. To most members of society, especially during a war, news is valuable as building community and as providing information about the fate of loved ones.[48] To the public, therefore, news is primarily valuable in noneconomic ways. The disjunction between the public's noneconomic modes of valuing news and the news services' strictly economic valuation of news weighed on the majority.

This disjunction may have caused alarm because it threatened to upset the requirement that all parties value the news in terms of its market price. The majority feared that if it recognized the existence of a property right in news in a case where both parties did, in fact, value it economically, the Court might later be required to uphold that right in a case against a party that valued news solely in noneconomic ways. This would violate the requirement that a good cannot be property where the primary value of the good to any party is noneconomic. Such a case could occur if, for example, a news service, relying on its property right, refused to release news to which it had exclusive access. In order to be consistent, the Court would be forced to recognize the news agency's property right in the news even though the public, from whom the news was being withheld, valued the news in noneconomic ways. On the other hand, a refusal to consider the award of a property right where both parties agreed that the only interest at stake was economic would create uncertainty. Parties would not know, in the future, what standards they would have to meet in order to satisfy a court that property rights ought to be granted. To get around this difficulty, the majority held that news, as between the two news services, was quasiproperty.[49] The majority refused to consider whether "any general and absolute property in news" existed. The decision to hold that news was equivalent to property, but only for the purposes of the dispute between INS and AP, allowed the majority to hold that AP had satisfied the requirement that both parties value the news in terms of its market price while preserving a future court's ability, in a different case with different parties, to hold that this hurdle had not been traversed.

In his dissent, Justice Brandeis rejected the majority's implicit assertion that the interests of the news services could be analyzed in isolation from the public interest.[50] In doing so, he reformulated the requirement that the parties value the contested good primarily in terms of market price to hold that the only significant value inhering in the contested good must be economic before the courts ought to consider the grant of a property right. Where noneconomic,[51] as opposed to strictly economic, values affect a good, Justice Brandeis held, the Court should not award an unqualified right of ownership.[52] Further, where, as in the case of news, the noneconomic interests were "omnipresent," the courts should defer any decision as to the allocation of rights to the legislature. Justice Brandeis wrote that, given the complexity of the interests involved with news, the legislature was better able than the courts to establish boundaries to any right to news and better able to enforce such limitations.[53]

Sowing and Reaping: Raising Economics to the Moral Plane

Having determined that the primary value of news—at least for the purposes of the dispute between INS and AP—was its market price, the majority turned to the issue of whether AP ought to have a property right in the news. At this point in its analysis, the majority introduced a powerful argument in favor of granting such a right, powerful both because it is strongly emotive and because later judges have found it convincing.[54] The majority's argument rests on an analogy between the good under discussion, here news, and the sowing and reaping of wheat. Whoever sows wheat, the majority asserted, ought to be able to reap the wheat. It is only just, the argument holds, that he or she who has planted and cared for the wheat over many months ought to be able to harvest the wheat when mature and sell it for a profit. Any intruder who, just as the wheat matures, gathers the wheat and sells it for his or her own benefit has offended against the farmer who cultivated the wheat. By analogy, the majority contended, AP, which had collected and packaged the news at the expense of both labor and money, was entitled to reap the benefits of its efforts. INS, playing the part of interloper, harvested the news at the very moment that AP was about to sell it. In so doing, the majority concluded, INS acted unjustly.[55]

The analogy between news and wheat, while at first blush forceful, is actually misleading. First, as others have noted,[56] wheat and news are quite different goods. Because wheat is a tangible good, possession by one person precludes possession by another; news, on the other hand, being intangible, can be possessed by several unrelated people simultaneously. That is, several unconnected individuals can make use of the news without interfering in the use made of it by others.[57] Thus, unlike the case of wheat, one should not assume that there ought to be but one unique possessor of news. A second aspect of the analogy reveals a more fundamental difficulty. The force of the analogy between wheat and news derives, obviously, from the feeling that the intruder did something wrong in harvesting the wheat. But the reason we feel this way has less to do with the fact that the farmer had sowed and cared for the wheat than with the presumption that the farmer possessed the land upon which the wheat was grown.[58] What the intruder did in harvesting the wheat was to interfere with the farmer's possession of the land and with the farmer's use of the land. To see this, consider the example of a farmer who sows wheat on a neighbor's land. Although, in such a case, we might be sympathetic to the farmer should the neighbor decide to harvest and sell the wheat, we are unlikely to feel that any injustice had been perpetrated.[59] The farmer's investment of time and labor in the cultivation of the wheat is not sufficient to create a property right; the law only grants such rights to farmers who have some possessory right to land upon which the wheat is grown. By punishing the intruder for gathering the wheat, the law is actually protecting the farmer's possessory interest in the land and the farmer's right to use the land. Whatever power the analogy between wheat and news possesses is, therefore, more a testament to the cultural and legal importance of land than to any general principle of law based on sowing and reaping. In sum, it is simply not the case that the investment of time and labor is sufficient to create property rights; there are too many counterexamples to this proposition for it to be true.

If sowing does not necessarily create the right to reap, there is a mystery of sorts to be explained. As stated, the judges in the majority in *INS* were not the only ones who succumbed to the power of the sowing and reaping analogy; later judges and courts addressing the issue of proprietary interests in intangibles have found the analogy convincing. If the proposition is so obviously fallacious, the courts' invocations of it must be explained. One source of the proposition's force may be its seeming similarity to Locke's labor theory of property.[60] Roughly, Locke stated that the individual who mixed his or her labor with a previously unowned good became the owner of that good. It is unnecessary to descend into a critique of Locke's theory[61] in order to undermine the analogy between the sowing and reaping argument and Locke's understanding of property. Locke was concerned with the creation of property rights in goods which were capable of being subject to such rights; his labor theory does not tell us which goods fall into this category. The question before courts such as the Court in INS was whether property rights ought to exist in the intangible goods before them. That is, one can invoke Locke—assuming one accepts his theory—only after having determined that property rights ought to exist in a particular good. One cannot invoke Locke's labor theory of property to determine the category of goods in which such rights ought to exist. It is not enough, therefore, that AP labored to collect news; the question that must first be answered is whether anyone ought to own the news. AP's efforts carry moral weight, if at all, only if this question has been answered in the affirmative.

One explanation for the mysterious reliance on the sowing and reaping argument is that the majority in INS simply missed a step in its analysis. In other words, the majority simply assumed that news could be the subject of property rights. A more careful reading of the majority opinion leads, however, to another conclusion. Hidden within its sowing and reaping argument, the majority revealed that property rights to news must be accepted in order to promote trade in news, and that the promotion of trade is the primary goal of property law.[62] The majority's argument is as follows. News has a short life span as a commercial product. Because of this short life span, individuals and organizations must continually collect and disseminate news. Given the large expense in labor, money, and skill involved in the collection and transmission of news, such individuals and organizations will only collect and disseminate news if they are provided with the economic incentive to do so.[63] This economic incentive is provided by the market value of news.[64] If organizations such as INS are permitted to wrest this exchange value from those who have invested capital and labor in the collection of news, then no one, in the future, will be willing to make such an investment. Ultimately, while the demand for news will be high, the supply of news will become negligible. Although the price of news will rise, there will be no similar rise in the production of news. The market will, therefore, fail.

The majority, in reaching the decision to award AP a proprietary interest in news, eschewed a direct consideration of the nonmarket values inhering in news gathering and transmission.[65] That is, the majority did not directly investigate whether the noneconomic values implicated in news gathering and transmission would be furthered or hindered by according AP a property right in the news. In fact, after briefly noting that news is socially important, the majority did not again discuss the matter.[66] The majority's behavior in this regard may be a reflection of its assumption that the promotion of a healthy market in news furthered, albeit indirectly, all values inhering in news. This is so, this assumption holds, because every person will attach a price to how she or he values news. The market price of news will come to reflect all these values. Since every way of valuing news will be represented in the marketplace, there is no need, the argument continues, for an explicit evaluation of the societal values inhering in news.

By appearing to reward effort, however, the analogy to sowing and reaping wheat countered the coldness of the majority's market analysis. The analogy effectively elevated the decision to let the market rank societal values inhering in news to the moral plane. In the result, the majority was left in the enviable position of both side-stepping a difficult moral decision—the ranking of values inhering in news— and justifying this side-stepping by invoking moral considerations. Never mind that this particular moral justification was more apparent than real.

Justice Brandeis saw through the majority's forced analogy between news and wheat. He stated that the fact that an individual had labored on a good does not ensure that the law will regard that good as the property of that individual.[67] Having recognized the hollowness of the sowing and reaping analogy, he turned to the real basis upon which the majority determined that AP had a proprietary interest in the news: the promotion of trade in news. Justice Brandeis argued that, far from increasing trade in news, the award of a property right to AP would hinder the dissemination of news. The grant of a property right in news to AP would, in effect, grant AP a monopoly in news. Such a monopoly ran counter to the public interest, Justice Brandeis held. Since, as he pointed out, as many as half of the newspaper readers in the United States relied on news agencies other than AP for their news, if AP did not share its news, a large proportion of the public would be without news concerning the war.[68] Trade in news is, therefore, enhanced, according to this analysis, by withholding property rights to news.

The argument canvassed by the majority, that the accord of property rights enhances trade, and the counterargument formulated by Justice Brandeis, that property rights create monopolies that stifle trade, together form the substance of current debates over the ownership of hitherto unowned intangible goods, assuming that the parties value the contested good in terms of price. The market analysis employed by those seeking property protection emphasizes the salutary effect on trade when individuals are rewarded for their efforts. The market analysis brandished by those opposed to the award of property rights highlights the trade-inhibiting effect of granting a monopoly over the use of a good. The sophistication of the analysis varies from case to case—although, in general, the analysis tends to be fairly crude—but its presence is the leitmotif of any drama centered on the recognition of new property rights in intangibles.

The two-step analysis illustrated in *INS* is repeated, in some form, in all the property cases analyzed in the next several chapters. It is thus worth summarizing. The first step is the determination that all parties value the contested good in terms of its market price. In *INS*, the majority had little difficulty making this determination but was afraid that, in a future case between a news agency and the public, the public interest in news would be noneconomic. Because of this desire to avoid being forced to enforce a news agency's property claim to news against the public, the majority held that news would only be considered property as between news agencies. Justice Brandeis, dissenting, disagreed with the majority's solution. He held that because a potential future party, the public, valued news in noneconomic ways, news ought not to be considered property even as between INS and AP. The second step in the analysis led to a similar disagreement between the majority and the dissent. The majority held that property rights to news were essential to ensure continued trade in news. Without an economic incentive to produce news, the majority contended, no one would collect it. Thus, there would be no news to trade. Justice Brandeis countered that the award of a property right in news merely created a monopoly in news. Such a monopoly hindered trade in news and left a sizable proportion of the public without prompt access to important information about the war.

The majority's faith in the market to rank all values inhering in a good parallels the opinions in *Stanley v. Columbia Broadcasting System, Inc.*[69] and *Murray v. National Broadcasting Co.*,[70] examined earlier in this chapter. In both of these cases, instead of deliberating upon the various ways in which a program idea may have been valuable, the judges felt their role was simply to ensure that there was a functioning market in these ideas. This market would do the magic of ranking each of the ways program ideas could be valued. In order to secure a functioning market in program ideas, the judges sought to maximize the number of these ideas in existence. They did so by providing an economic incentive to create new goods: the allocation of property rights. At the same time, the judges attempted to prevent the creation of monopolies of ideas, which stifle development, by withholding property protection from abstract ideas and discoveries.

The danger inherent in the majority's and the *Stanley* and *Murray* courts' reliance on the market to allocate rights of control over goods is that the courts will allocate these rights without reference to the noneconomic modes of valuation that may inhere in those goods. That is, while an allocation on this basis may indeed maximize the economic value of a good, it may ignore or actually harm the noneconomic values inhering in the good. The market answer to this danger is that the market does, albeit indirectly—through the determination of market price—allocate goods on the basis of all values inhering in the good. But this answer is premised on our ability to translate noneconomic modes of valuation into a market price and our ability to rank these market prices against each other. While I discuss these premises in greater detail in chapters 8 and 9, I note here that it is far from clear whether either of these premises can be defended.

Since many of the ways we value human biological materials are noneconomic, if these premises underlying property discourse cannot be sustained, then allocating rights of control over human biological materials within this discourse may encourage only the economic values inhering in these materials, to the detriment of noneconomic values. Thus we will encourage those who desire to use, to sell, or to consume human biological materials at the expense of those who value these materials in terms of dignity, respect, and sharing.

The decisions in *International News Service*, *Stanley*, and *Murray* resulted from disputes between individuals or companies who only valued the news and program ideas for their commercial potential. One could, therefore, explain the decisions in these cases as simply dealing with those values advanced by the parties; in other cases, where the parties value the disputed good in accordance with noneconomic modes of valuation, one could argue, the courts will allocate rights of control based on those modes of valuation. In order to test this challenge to my analysis, and ultimately demonstrate that even where the disputants value a good in noneconomic ways the courts nevertheless allocate rights of control as if only economic modes of valuation counted, I review, in the next three chapters, court decisions in which the disputants valued the disputed good increasingly in accordance with noneconomic modes of valuation.

The cases that I discuss in the next three chapters, although not directly related to human biological materials, each involves a decision whether to apply property discourse to a good that, prior to that case, had not been subject to that discourse. Each case presents, therefore, parallels with the present situation in which human biological materials are largely exempt from property discourse but may soon become the subject matter of property law disputes. How the courts have treated other goods that have become subject to property discourse provides the best indication of how courts are likely to deal with human biological materials. This is because, as discussed in chapter 1, the process of legal reasoning is largely historical, with past decisions determining, to a large extent, the answer to any legal question. While radical change is, in theory, possible, the constraints in the manner in which legal decisions are made strongly militate against any large change in the short term.

In the next chapter, I commence the foray into the nature of property discourse by examining claims by inventors to goods that they value economically, although others may value them in other ways. Chapter 5 examines the claims of public personalities to their personae. These individuals rely exclusively on the economic value of their personae in claiming a property right to their personae despite their often stronger noneconomic attachments to it. Finally, chapter 6 focuses on two cases in which the parties' primary interest in the contested good is noneconomic. In one case the party convinces the court that this noneconomic interest is, in reality, economically valuable and thus wins a property right. In the other case, the party musters a strong moral claim to the contested good but loses because the party is unable to translate this moral claim into a market price.

In chapter 7, once I have completed my analysis of property discourse, I examine some of the ways in which we value human biological materials and conclude that most of these ways are noneconomic in nature. For those who would rather skip the detailed analysis of property discourse that I present in the next three chapters, chapter 7 signals the return to our discussion of human biological materials.

4

The Discourse of Discovery

It was on a dreary night of November, that I beheld
the accomplishment of my toils. With an anxiety that almost
amounted to agony, I collected the instruments of life around
me, that I might infuse a spark of being into the lifeless thing
that lay at my feet. It was already one in the morning; the rain
pattered dismally against the panes, and my candle was nearly
burnt out, when, by the glimmer of the half-extinguished light,
I saw the dull yellow eye of the creature open; it breathed
hard, and a convulsive motion agitated its limbs.

How can I describe my emotions at this catastrophe, or
how delineate the wretch whom with such infinite pains and
care I had endeavoured to form.[1]

One need not be an academic in order to ponder the future of biotechnological research and the values inhering in human biological materials. Literature and film have long explored the implications of technological development on society and on our understanding of
humanity. Frankenstein's monster, the creation of biotechnological
research using human biological materials, has a secure home in Western imagination.[2] The monster illustrates, in its film and literary incar-
nations, both the fear that technology robs us of our humanity[3] and
the belief that technology itself is not evil; it is only some of the
purposes to which it is put that are diabolic.[4] The Frankenstein story's
continued ability to haunt us—there are new film versions of it made
every few years[5]—reveals society's ambivalence toward technological
development.

Property law, by contrast, is not ambivalent about technological
development. Patent law, that part of property law dealing with new
technological innovation, is expressly designed to encourage such
development.[6] Courts assume that such innovation benefits society

not only through the introduction of new products, but through increased employment and the general betterment of the lives of the citizenry.[7] The themes so prevalent in film and literature—concern over the impact of new technologies on our culture, self-understanding, health, and environment—find no counterpart in patent-law discourse.

In this chapter I continue our excursion into property discourse, but with the goal of determining how courts and those who argue before them approach goods that theretofore had not been considered property and thus had not been the subject matter of property discourse. The object of this analysis is to determine how courts and legal practitioners are likely to treat human biological materials when disputants present their claims to rights of control over these materials to the courts. My aim in this chapter and in chapters 5 and 6 is to examine the application of property discourse to new kinds of goods and not to analyze how courts currently approach human biological materials. This examination of property discourse will lead, in chapters 8 and 9, to a discussion of the likely consequences of applying this discourse to human biological materials.

This survey of court decisions is important to our understanding of property discourse. While most individuals within society do not directly participate in property discourse as practiced in the courtroom, what courts say about property rights nevertheless has significant effects on all of our lives. When a court recognizes a property right in a good, that recognition is binding on all members of society. That is, once a court holds that a certain individual has the right to control a particular good, all of us are obliged to respect that holding.

Since the object of property discourse is to allocate rights of control, we all have a vested interest in how this discourse, whether or not we directly participate in it, will be applied to human biological materials. If, through this discourse, courts or Congress allocate rights of control over these materials in a way that does harm to the way that we, in this society, actually value these materials, then it may prove difficult to right this harm later.

The analysis in chapter 3 began the argument that when courts allocate rights of control over a good, they do so exclusively on the basis of economic ways of valuing the disputed good. As stated in that chapter, courts narrow their focus to economic modes of valuation not out of any disregard for noneconomic modes of valuation, but because they assume that all modes of valuation are translatable into a market price. Therefore, the assumption continues, if the courts ensure that the market functions fairly and openly, the market will, in turn, ensure that property rights will be allocated to those individuals who most value the good, as reflected in the price that they are willing to pay for it. This assumption is implicit in property discourse and goes unchallenged in property cases for the simple reason that disputants find it easier and more successful to frame their arguments in accordance with established lines of reasoning than to challenge the assumptions behind property discourse.

We do not, fortunately, have to adopt this procrustean solution with respect to human biological materials, as these materials have not yet been made the subject matter of property discourse. Before disputants present their cases to the courts or to Congress, we can ask how property discourse can be expected to affect the ways we value human biological materials. Before we can speculate on how property discourse will affect how we value these materials, however, we need to establish which modes of valuation we encourage and which we discourage through property discourse.

This chapter examines two series of patent law cases to illustrate that the thesis developed in the last chapter, that courts look exclusively at a good's economic value in determining whether the good ought to be the subject of property rights, applies in full force to patent law. Each of the two series of cases focuses on one of the two most revolutionary technologies of the late twentieth century: computers and biotechnology. The issue before the courts in both series is whether the products of these two technologies are patentable. Because computers and biotechnology represent a fundamental break from previous technologies, the courts adjudicating these claims could not reason by analogy; they were forced to work from first principles. This, coupled with the fact that most of the cases are of relatively recent vintage, makes these series highly inviting to analysis.

Patent Law

By statute, a discovery is patentable only if it is useful, novel, and nonobvious.[8] Roughly speaking, a discovery is useful when it results in a manufactured good that can be sold on the market.[9] In practice, however, courts spend little time examining an invention for utility;[10] rather, they assume that no one would bother to patent an invention that had no "use."[11] The novelty requirement precludes the award of patent rights in a good that has already been manufactured or has already been described in the literature. The nonobviousness requirement states that only those inventions that are not obvious to a person of ordinary skill in the relevant field of knowledge using publicly available material are patentable.[12]

The courts understand patent law to be premised on the promotion of commerce rather than on the promotion of noneconomic values such as self-development or community. Consider, for example, the judicial definition of the usefulness requirement. The United States Supreme Court has held that a discovery that is "useful" only in the sense that it is of scientific interest—such as a new compound health researchers wish to investigate for tumor-inhibiting effects—does not qualify as being useful under the statute.[13] The implication of the Court's argument is that to grant patent rights in an invention before it is reduced to a marketable good would be to remove the economic incentive necessary to encourage researchers to find marketable uses for the invention. Usefulness, under this definition, depends entirely on an invention's market price. Except to the extent that they impinge on this price, an invention's noneconomic characteristics—its aesthetic, safety, and inspirational qualities, for example—are irrelevant to the judicial determination of whether patent rights ought to attach to that invention.

The conclusion that an invention's economic value is central to the determination of whether patent rights attach to that invention emerges from a consideration of three lines of analysis that the courts undertake in arriving at such determinations. First, courts ask whether the grant of a monopoly, in the form of a patent right, is likely to stifle further invention or whether it is likely to encourage new discovery by providing an economic incentive to invest in research and development. Behind this line of analysis is the view that patent law represents a balance between two economic forces.[14] The first of these forces is free trade in goods. The competition implicit in free trade not only ensures the efficient production of goods but provides the backdrop against which the second force, the monopolistic one, acts. Competition so reduces the profit that can be made from freely traded goods that many individuals are unwilling to invest in researching and developing new products. This is where the monopolistic force comes into play. Because of the small profit to be made from freely traded goods, individuals are anxious to win monopoly powers in order to garner the potentially large profits to be made from them. Patent law relies on this anxiety to increase the stock of goods available to the public by granting monopoly powers to individuals who successfully research and develop new goods. Monopolies are not, however, without their drawbacks. If granted too freely over too wide an area of endeavor, monopolies hinder inventive activity by preventing those who would advance a technology from undertaking research and from bringing cheaper and better versions of the technology to market. Thus, neither the force of free trade nor the force of monopoly is sufficient on its own to ensure the vigorous development of inventions. When the monopolistic and free trade forces are correctly balanced, however, the rate of technological development is maximized.

This first line of analysis, that monopolistic and free trade forces must balance to ensure maximum invention, is analogous to the second hurdle to the grant of property rights set out in chapter 3. That chapter identified two hurdles that a property claimant must traverse to receive a property right. First is the requirement that all parties to a dispute must value the contested good in terms of its market value. Second is the requirement that the grant of property rights must enhance, rather than hinder, trade in the good. In their patent-law decisions, courts assume that parties value inventions in terms of their market price because the courts believe that no one would be willing to expend time and money to develop an invention and to prosecute and defend a patent unless there were economic rewards for doing so.[15] Thus, courts assume that the first hurdle to the award of property rights has been negotiated. The second hurdle, that the award of property rights enhance trade in the contested good, remains to be cleared. Debate over whether a property claimant has traversed this hurdle occupies the bulk of the decisions that this chapter examines.

The second line of analysis followed in deciding whether to grant patent rights is the determination of whether the good in question—for example, a computer program or a biological organism—is or is analogous to a phenomenon of nature.[16] If it is, the courts hold that it ought to be freely available. Behind this line of inquiry are two moral propositions: that what nature has provided ought to be shared by all and that one can only appropriate what one has created out of nature's bounty. This argument serves much the same function as did the sowing and reaping argument in *International News Service v. Associated Press*:[17] it provides a moral veneer for what is, essentially, an economic decision to award or to withhold patent rights.[18] This is so because the determination that a discovery is a "phenomenon of nature" turns out to be a decision that the monopolization of the discovery would impede further invention.[19]

The third line of analysis displaying the centrality of economic value in the decision whether to award patent rights is the determination of which values inhering in an invention are open to judicial scrutiny and which are not. Courts hold themselves institutionally competent to explicitly consider certain values inhering in a discovery, namely economic ones, and incompetent to consider other values, namely noneconomic ones. The latter values can only be addressed, the courts suggest, by the legislature. This admission of judicial incompetence does not, however, prevent the courts from adjudicating patent-law disputes; instead, the courts limit themselves to a consideration of exclusively economic factors in deciding such cases. In so doing, the courts assume that whatever noneconomic values inhere in an invention will be appropriately ranked through market processes. Thus, the assumption continues, so long as the courts ensure that the market in inventions is healthy, the market itself will ensure that noneconomic ways of valuing inventions are properly considered. The market accomplishes this task, as discussed in chapters 1 and 3, by allocating an invention to that individual who is willing to pay the most for it. Since the price an individual is willing to pay for an invention is assumed to be directly proportional to the strength of the way in which that individual values the invention, the market ensures that the invention ends up in the hands of the individual who values it most.

If the label "property" represents the legal conclusion that a good is valuable,[20] then, by holding themselves incompetent to consider noneconomic values inhering in inventions, the courts demonstrate that value means only economic value. Thus, this third line of analysis, more clearly than the other two, supports the thesis that the only relevant value in the determination of whether a discovery is to be made subject to patent law is the discovery's market price.

Patents to Computer Software

Computer technology differs from other technologies primarily due to the fact that a significant part of what makes the technology important is intangible. Without this intangible component—computer programs and algorithms—computers cannot operate. Programs consist of lists of instructions that a computer, using other programs, translates into a tangible, usable form. Programs can be written at various levels of abstraction, from machine language, at the least abstract end of the spectrum, to a formal computer language, such as LISP or C, at the other. Computers translate abstract computer languages into less abstract ones and then translate the result into machine-readable code. The translation process from higher language to lower language and from lower language into machine code is dependent on both the physical computer and the translating programs used. Thus, a program written in an abstract computer language could translate into any of a number of different sets of machine code.

An algorithm is similar to a computer program, except that it is written in a human language and must be translated into a computer language by a programmer. Given the wide choice of computer languages available and programmers' personal idiosyncracies, a given algorithm can be translated into many different programs written in many different computer languages. Since each such program can be translated into myriad sets of machine code, depending on the computer and the translating program used, a given algorithm could be translated into any of an extremely large number of physical representations.

Computer programs and algorithms can be thought of as literary plots. Just as the story of two star-crossed lovers can lead to such diverse productions as *Romeo and Juliet* and *West Side Story*, so an algorithm can lead to many different computer programs which, in turn, can be represented differently in different computers. With each layer of abstraction, from programs written in machine language to programs written in abstract computer languages to algorithms, the number of physical representations corresponding to the program or algorithm increases in much the same way as the number of possible plays increases when one increases the generality of a plot from lovers belonging to two hostile clans to lovers whose love is thwarted by forces outside of their control to simply lovers.[21]

The fact that computer programs and algorithms are intangible constructions with many tangible representations makes their subjugation to patent law difficult. Should programs and algorithms be subject to patent rights, a right to a particular program or algorithm would encompass all the myriad physical representations of that program or algorithm. Thus, if one were to grant a patent right in an algorithm, one would be simultaneously granting such a right in all possible computer programs, written in any computer language, that implemented that algorithm. Granting a patent right in such algorithms, just as granting a property right in all possible stories based on the plot of star-crossed lovers, would be tantamount to granting a monopoly power over a very large area of endeavor. Such wideranging monopoly powers are likely to upset the careful balance between the economic forces of monopoly and free trade that the courts believe underlie patent law.

This section of the chapter looks at three cases decided by the United States Supreme Court that raise the issue of whether algorithms and programs are patentable. All three cases illustrate the central role that economics plays in deciding whether a good is to be made subject to patent law. Further, these cases demonstrate that the size of this role has increased over time.

Benson: The First Attempt

Gottschalk v. Benson[22] represents the Court's first attempt to determine whether computer programs and algorithms should be subject to patent law. Benson devised an algorithm for converting binary-coded decimal numbers (called BCD numerals) into their pure binary equivalents.[23] From this algorithm, a specific set of instructions could be written to suit the particular computer on which it was to run. Benson claimed patent protection for the algorithm, no matter how and where it was used.

In refusing to grant Benson's claim to a patent in the algorithm, the Court pointed to the wide monopoly his claim entailed. The Court understood that Benson's claim was not restricted to a specific physical representation of the algorithm but to all such representations.[24] The large scope of Benson's claim would entirely preempt a whole range of activity, the Court held, including efforts to find novel ways of using the algorithm. Patent rights only attach to an invention, the Court continued, where it has been reduced to a specific form. Since Benson's claim encompassed all physical forms of the algorithm, it was too broad to be protected under patent law. Given the scope of Benson's claim, the Court concluded that granting a patent would not promote inventive activity; it would stifle it.

The *Benson* Court bolstered its conclusion that patent rights ought not to be granted in algorithms by holding that algorithms are analogous to phenomena of nature, the latter being defined as the "basic tools of scientific and technological work."[25] Future innovation depends, the Court held, on the ability of researchers and investors to make use of such phenomena in order to create new and better goods. Monopoly powers in such phenomena, in the form of patent rights, interfere with innovation by blocking access to such phenomena.[26] Phenomena of nature must, therefore, remain subject to free trade; otherwise, innovation will decrease and there will be fewer goods to trade. Because algorithms stand in the same position relative to computer science as do phenomena of nature to the physical sciences, the argument concludes, algorithms ought to be freely traded.

Notice the parallels between the arguments that the grant of patent rights in algorithms would upset the delicate balance between monopolistic and free trade forces and the argument that algorithms are analogous to phenomena of nature—in that algorithms are laws of nature, expressed mathematically, awaiting discovery by a mathematician—and thus ought not to be owned by anyone. Phenomena of nature ought not to be subject to patent rights, the Court held, because to do so would upset the balance between monopolistic and free trade forces that underlies patent law. In so holding, the Court merged the two arguments into one. This is odd, however, because the two arguments are quite distinct. The phenomena of nature argument asserts the moral proposition that nature's bounty belongs to all;[27] the balance argument relies on strictly economic considerations. Without its moral underpinning, the phenomena of nature argument would be circular, for it would fail to explain why nature's bounty ought to belong to everyone instead of to whomever first came along and took it. The moral underpinning is thus Lockean in nature. It holds that God intended people to make use of the Earth and its resources and that, once a person has used a resource, that person becomes its owner.[28] Phenomena of nature are different, according to this view, from other goods because they enable us to carry out divine purposes.

On the other hand, the argument that monopoly control of algorithms unacceptably stifles inventive activity is strictly economic. It entails no moral precept and demands from us no moral response. It is, in this respect, very different from the phenomena of nature argument. It further differs from the latter argument in that it is based on empirical evidence. Our conclusion with respect to whether patent rights ought to attach to a good, as far as this economic argument is concerned, is subject to change should new data become available. The conclusion of the phenomena of nature argument, that such phenomena ought not to be subject to patent rights, is not subject to change irrespective of the discovery of new evidence. Thus, while it may be true that both the balancing of forces and the phenomena of nature arguments lead to the same conclusion with respect to computer algorithms, there is no guarantee that they will coincide with respect to other goods.

The *Benson* Court's willingness to view the balancing of forces and the phenomena of nature arguments as equivalent tells us something fundamental about how courts value inventions within patent law. The Court understood the phenomena of nature argument to state an economic proposition with a moral twist. This proposition is that inventive activity ought to be encouraged and that this is best accomplished by encouraging the free use of phenomena of nature. The moral twist is that this reliance on the market is mandated by God, or, more generally, by a moral principle—that all of us ought to have equal access to the natural environment in order to make our own way in life. The moral basis for this twist is, however, illusory. It is based on the view that phenomena of nature are inviolate and ought to be treated as such. Once one subjugates such phenomena, however, to market principles, they are no longer inviolate. That is, once one replaces market criteria for respect of the inviolate, the phenomena of nature argument loses its moral imperative. It becomes simply shorthand for the market conclusion that the grant of patent rights in abstract goods stifles inventive activity.

Although the phenomena of nature argument loses its moral force when equated with the balancing of forces argument, it still looks like a moral argument and thus appears to carry moral weight. This may explain why the Court in *Benson* relied on it when the balancing argument was sufficient to justify its conclusion that algorithms are not patentable. Just as in the case of the sowing and reaping argument in *International News Service v. Associated Press*,[29] the phenomena of nature argument provided a moral front for an economic conclusion.[30]

The Court's final ground for rejecting Benson's claim to a patent right in his algorithm was the judicial competency argument. The Court stated that the grant of patent rights in algorithms raised policy questions to which it was "not competent to speak."[31] The Court held that only Congress had the resources and the institutional mandate to consider and balance these policy questions. It may be noted that this lack of competency did not deter the Court from engaging in a serious discussion of the likely economic effects of granting patent rights in algorithms; the Court held itself incompetent only in respect of an evaluation of the noneconomic factors touching on inventions.

Elucidating the Phenomena of Nature Argument

The United States Supreme Court again examined the issue of the patentability of computer programs and algorithms in *Parker v. Flook*.[32] The decision in *Flook* is more an elucidation of the phenomena of nature argument used in *Benson* than a clear discussion of the goals of patent law. In *Flook*, the Court attempted to differentiate between an unpatentable phenomenon of nature and a patentable process that relied on such a phenomenon. In drawing this distinction, the Court demonstrated the distance it had put between the phenomena of nature argument and the argument's moral core.

Flook formulated an algorithm to calculate whether certain chemical reactions had run awry. He sought patent protection for this algorithm as used in conjunction with the catalytic conversion of hydrocarbons; his patent claim did not cover other uses of the algorithm. To use the algorithm, an operator had to independently determine a margin of safety, a weighting factor, and other variables connected with a particular reaction. With these variables and the algorithm, the operator could calculate whether the reaction was behaving in an acceptable manner.

Relying on the decision in *Benson*, the *Flook* Court asserted that algorithms, being analogous to phenomena of nature, ought not to be patentable.[33] Algorithms, like phenomena of nature, comprise part of the storehouse of knowledge open to all inventors. Inventors can lay claim only to what they create from this knowledge. Thus patent law grants rights in discoveries that concretize such knowledge in a useful form but not in the underlying knowledge itself. In determining whether a patent claim is valid, the Court held, the underlying knowledge ought to be treated as part of the prior art, whether or not this knowledge had been previously known. The Court should only grant a patent right in the discovery if the discovery is novel and useful without this knowledge.

Flook claimed that his catalytic conversion process was patentable because it was an application of an algorithm and not an algorithm itself. The Court rejected this argument, holding that, despite its appearance, Flook's claim was to the underlying algorithm. The limitation Flook placed on his patent claim, that the claim only apply to the use of the algorithm in conjunction with the catalytic conversion of hydrocarbons, was arbitrary.[34] The Court stated that merely limiting the scope of one's patent claim to a subset of the possible uses of an algorithm was insufficient to meet the requirements of patent law.[35] Only those programs or algorithms that, by their very nature, are limited to specific applications are patentable.[36] The limitation of Flook's claim to catalytic conversions was thus characterized as an afterthought on an algorithm of general application.

Just as in *Benson*, the Court buttressed its rejection of Flook's claims by holding that the courts were not competent to evaluate the many "[d]ifficult questions of policy concerning the kinds of programs that may be appropriate for patent protection and the form and duration of such protection."[37] These policy questions, the Court held, could only be answered by Congress. The Court concluded that it ought, therefore, to defer any decision over the patentability of programs and algorithms to Congress. Again, as in *Benson*, the Court's self-stated lack of competence with respect to resolving policy issues did not deter it from holding that algorithms ought not to be patentable for economic reasons.

The *Flook* Court was far from clear about why phenomena of nature, as opposed to other discoveries, ought not to be patentable. While the Court hinted that there was a moral justification behind the phenomena of nature argument, it never explicitly stated what this justification might be.[38] The Court simply acted on the belief that there is a difference between phenomena of nature and all other discoveries and that some practical rule was needed to differentiate between the two. In short, the Court in *Flook* began to use the phenomena of nature argument independently of its moral core.

Refocusing the Phenomena of Nature Argument

In its decision in *Diamond v. Diehr*,[39] the United States Supreme Court completed the process of separating the phenomena of nature argument from its moral roots. It accomplished this by focusing the argument away from the debate over whether certain discoveries are off-bounds to patent law toward the debate over whether a particular invention is too abstract, in the sense of covering too wide an area of endeavor, to be patentable. By refocusing the use to which the phenomena of nature argument was put, the Court effectively converted the argument from a statement of moral principle to an expression of economic concern over the scope of monopoly powers.

Diehr sought to patent a process for molding raw, uncured synthetic rubber into cured precision products. Diehr added to the prior art of molding and curing rubber by introducing a computer to repeatedly monitor the temperature within the mold and to calculate, using this information, when the rubber was cured. The computer would then instruct the mold to open. Diehr did not claim to have added any new physical steps to the curing process; his only claim to novelty was the introduction of a computer to continuously update the curing time.

The characterization of Diehr's invention was central to the outcome in the case.[40] The majority held that Diehr had invented a new process to cure rubber using computers.[41] This contrasts markedly with the Court's characterization of the inventions in *Benson* and *Flook*. There, the Court had held that only the algorithms were novel; the processes to which the algorithms were added were not. Thus the Court, in those cases, found that Benson's and Flook's patent claims were limited to the algorithms and did not extend to the underlying processes. This is especially apparent in *Flook*, where the Court firmly distinguished between Flook's algorithm and the underlying process, the catalytic conversion of hydrocarbons.[42] The *Diehr* Court, by contrast, sympathetically viewed Diehr's algorithm as being a constituent part of a manufacturing process and not simply an addition to it. On this view, Diehr had invented not only an algorithm but a new process to cure synthetic rubber.

The dissent in *Diehr* disagreed with the majority's characterization of the invention. The dissent wrote that Diehr's invention was no more than an algorithm. It held that although this algorithm could be used to cure synthetic rubber, Diehr did not invent the underlying process.[43] In fact, the dissent stated, Diehr's discovery was highly reminiscent of Flook's. Both discoveries centered around the calculation of a number, in Diehr's case the amount of time to cure rubber and in Flook's case a number corresponding to how well the catalytic conversion of hydrocarbons was functioning. These numbers were then used in existing processes to create exactly the same products as had always been manufactured using these processes. Therefore, the dissent concluded, just as the Court had rejected Flook's claim, it should also reject Diehr's.

The majority held that Diehr's invention was not a phenomenon of nature because it was not a lone algorithm but a process to transform a good into another state or thing.[44] While phenomena of nature, the majority conceded, cannot be the subject of a patent, an application of a phenomenon of nature is patentable. That is, a process that relies on a phenomenon of nature to transform a good into a different state or thing is patentable even though the phenomenon of nature itself is not patentable. Because Diehr's invention was a transforming process, the curing of synthetic rubber, and not an algorithm, Diehr was entitled to a patent over his invention.

This understanding of the phenomena of nature argument, that patents are not available in phenomena of nature themselves but are available in such phenomena to the extent that they are incorporated into concrete processes, exemplifies the break between the phenomena of nature argument and its moral origins. In its pure form, the phenomena of nature argument would preclude the award of patent rights in phenomena of nature in any form. Thus, in *Benson* and in *Flook*,[45] the Court rejected patent claims to algorithms even when incorporated into concrete processes. In these cases, phenomena of nature still carried the aura of being special or inviolate. In *Diehr*, by contrast, such phenomena had lost this aura. According to *Diehr*, the only difference between those goods that could be patented and those that could not was their degree of abstraction: the more abstract a good—for example, a pure mathematical formula—the less likely it could be patented; the more concrete a good—for example, a mathematical formula incorporated into a practical process—the more likely it was patentable.

Diehr represents the final stage of the movement begun in *Benson* and continued in *Flook* toward the disengagement of the phenomena of nature argument from its moral foundation. In this last stage, phenomena of nature no longer connote goods that are inviolate; rather, they are goods that are so abstract that the award of a patent right in them would undermine inventive activity. In this stage, economic principles have come to replace moral ones. Even the moral veneer, behind which the *Benson* and *Flook* Courts hid, disintegrated in *Diehr*. The *Diehr* majority, while recognizing the utility of the phenomena of nature argument, made no pretention that it was based on moral principle.[46]

The three cases discussed (*Benson*, *Flook*, and *Diehr*) illustrate that the courts value inventions (here computer programs and algorithms) with eyes clearly focused on their economic value. One alternative way of valuing programs as being inviolate goods, embodied within the phenomena of nature argument, did not find favor with the Court. Over time, the argument completely lost its moral force. Eventually, it came to stand for no more than the economic conclusion that patenting abstract goods would stifle inventive activity.

Patenting Living Organisms

The evolution of the phenomena of nature argument from one based on moral principle to one based on economic practicality repeats in the area of biotechnology. The remaining pages of this chapter examine two biotechnology cases from the United States Supreme Court dealing with patent claims to living organisms. In the first case, *Funk Brothers Seed Co. v. Kalo Inoculant Co.*,[47] the Court understood the phenomena of nature argument to stand for the proposition that certain goods cannot be owned because they are inviolate: that they were put on Earth for all to use equally. In the second case, *Diamond v. Chakrabarty*,[48] the Court abandoned this understanding. Instead of conceiving of the phenomena of nature argument as premised on moral principle, the Court perceived the argument to be based on economic principle. The Court's goal was to foster inventive activity, not to hold that certain goods were inviolate.

In *Funk Brothers*, the patent dispute centered on six species of bacteria from the genus *Rhizobium*. These bacteria infect the roots of leguminous plants, thereby enabling the plants to fix nitrogen from the air. Each of the six species infects the roots of different groups of leguminous plants. A farmer selects the appropriate species of *Rhizobium* for inoculation of the desired crop. The six species could not, however, be combined into a single inoculant because each inhibited the effect of the others. Therefore, farmers had to buy the particular species of bacteria that corresponded to their crop.

Bond discovered strains of each of the six species that did not display the normal inhibitory effect. He isolated these strains and mixed them together, forming a single inoculant that was effective on the entire range of leguminous plants. This single inoculant was easier to use and less expensive to store than the six individual inoculants, making it commercially valuable. Bond sought a patent for this discovery. The United States Supreme Court rejected his claim.

The Court held that bacteria are phenomena of nature and, as such, cannot be patented. Phenomena of nature, the Court stated, "are manifestations of laws of nature, free to all men and reserved to none."[49] No one, the Court emphasized, can claim a monopoly over such phenomena. Patent rights attach only to discoveries that arise out of the application of a phenomenon of nature. Unlike the Court in *Diehr*, however, the *Funk Brothers* Court did not mean by this that any application of a phenomenon of nature was patentable. In fact, the Court explicitly stated that it is not enough to transform a phenomenon of nature into a more useful form; the inventor must add something to it.

The Court acknowledged that Bond had created something new and useful. Bond not only discovered that there existed strains of *Rhizobia* that did not display a mutually inhibitive effect but packaged these strains in a commercially useful form. What Bond did not do, according to the Court, was to add anything to nature's handiwork. The six strains that Bond selected continued to carry out their natural function independent of him. Although Bond's development of a combined inoculant required skill, the Court held that it did not require invention.[50] Therefore, granting Bond a patent on his inoculant would be tantamount to the grant of a patent over "one of the ancient secrets of nature now discovered."

The Court's conclusion that the mere transformation of a phenomenon of nature into something new and useful is insufficient to gain patent rights contrasts markedly with the Court's later holding in *Diehr*. There, the Court held that exactly this type of transformation ensured patentability. Transformation of a phenomenon of nature into another state or thing ensured that the resulting invention was concrete and did not entail a stifling monopoly. Under the *Diehr* approach, there would have been no objection to the award of patent rights to Bond. After all, he had applied his scientific knowledge to transform naturally occurring bacteria into a new and usable form: a combined inoculant.

The *Funk Brothers* Court understood the phenomena of nature argument differently than did the *Diehr* Court. The *Funk Brothers* Court believed that phenomena of nature are special goods that cannot be owned. These goods are for all of humanity to share. No person can, therefore, claim more than the right to share in this beneficence. Certainly, no one is entitled to a monopoly over any part of it. Individuals are entitled, however, to own what they themselves create, even if their creation flows from the application of a phenomenon of nature. That is, individuals who add new goods—and not simply old goods in new forms—to humanity's storehouse of knowledge are entitled to patent rights. Bond, having only repackaged what nature had provided, was not entitled to these rights.

At bottom, the difference in approach between *Funk Brothers* and *Diehr* is that in the former a certain class of goods, phenomena of nature, are inviolate and cannot be owned while in the latter abstract goods, exemplified by phenomena of nature, cannot be patented because to do so would stifle inventive activity. *Funk Brothers* represents, in this interpretation, the high water mark of the moral power of the phenomena of nature argument[51] while *Diehr* represents its nadir.

Chakrabarty: Turning a Blind Eye to Noneconomic Values

The decision in *Diamond v. Chakrabarty*[52] refocused the phenomena of nature argument with respect to biotechnology in the same manner as *Diehr* had refocused the argument with respect to computer programs and algorithms. *Chakrabarty* went further than *Diehr* in one respect: in *Chakrabarty*, the Court bluntly refused to consider noneconomic ways of valuing inventions, holding itself competent to consider only the economic effects of granting or withholding patent rights. Because of this, *Chakrabarty* stands apart from the cases examined in this chapter in the forthrightness with which it tied patent rights to economic value.

Chakrabarty involved the creation, through genetic engineering, of a new bacterium that digests oil spills. Chakrabarty created this bacterium by introducing naturally occurring strands of genetic material into the cell of an existing bacterium. The added genetic material carried genes that enabled the bacterium to break down multiple components of crude oil. So far as was known, no naturally occurring bacterium carried out this function. Chakrabarty's discovery resembled Bond's discovery in *Funk Brothers* in significant ways. In both cases, the inventors selected previously existing genetic characteristics that permitted existing functions to be carried out in new ways. In both cases, the inventors mixed together a set of genes in a manner that would not occur in nature. In *Funk Brothers*, the mixture consisted of bacteria that would normally inhibit each other; in *Chakrabarty*, the mixture consisted of a set of genes that would not naturally be found in the same bacterium. The only real difference between the two cases is the form the inventions took: in *Funk Brothers*, naturally occurring bacteria in a nonnaturally occurring mixture; in *Chakrabarty*, a mixture of natural genes within a nonnaturally occurring bacterium. At bottom, both inventions amounted to no more than the repackaging of naturally occurring characteristics.

The United States Supreme Court held that Chakrabarty was entitled to a patent over his bacterium. The Court based its holding on a reworked version of the phenomena of nature argument and on judicial competency concerns. The Court stated that Congress intended that its patent laws be liberally interpreted so that "anything under the sun that is made by man" would be patentable.[53] Patent rights are essential, the Court held, to ensure inventive activity that will bolster the economy and lead to increased employment and better lives.[54]

Phenomena of nature represent an exception, according to the Court, from the general rule of patentability.[55] As befitting an exception, the Court accorded the phenomena of nature argument a narrower interpretation than had the Court in *Funk Brothers*. Phenomena of nature, the Court stated, include new minerals and plants and the laws of gravity and of relativity. Patentable goods differ, the Court held, from phenomena of nature in that they are the product of human ingenuity and research. Thus, the distinction the Court drew between phenomena of nature and patentable inventions hinged upon human intervention. Goods found in their natural form and abstract ideas cannot be owned, according to the Court, but goods that have been transformed from their natural state or ideas that have been put to a practical end are patentable. Phenomena of nature are not inviolate, therefore, as they were held to be in *Funk Brothers*, since they can easily be transformed into a patentable form. They remain, however, in the public domain as the raw material from which individuals are encouraged to invent.

The Court concluded that Chakrabarty's bacterium was not a phenomenon of nature. No naturally occurring bacterium carried out its function, and it was the result of human ingenuity and research. Consequently, the Court held that the bacterium ought to be patentable.

This conclusion is completely at odds with the decision in *Funk Brothers*. Under the Court's analysis in *Funk Brothers*, genetic characteristics are phenomena of nature and thus inviolate. An individual is not entitled to a patent over such characteristics merely by repackaging them. Chakrabarty did not invent the genetic code that enabled bacteria to digest crude oil; he only discovered the evidence of the code. Chakrabarty did not construct the bacterium into which he inserted the code; he found this bacterium in nature. In sum, Chakrabarty used well-known techniques to place naturally occurring genes within a naturally occurring bacterium. Although the resulting bacterium was not natural, neither was Bond's mixture of *Rhizobia*. Simply packaging phenomena of nature into a new and useful form is not enough, according to *Funk Brothers*, to win patent rights to such phenomena. In order to gain such rights, one must add something of one's own to the invention. This Chakrabarty did not do.

Although the *Chakrabarty* Court claimed to be adhering to the phenomena of nature argument as set out in *Funk Brothers*, it actually reformulated the argument to serve new purposes. In *Chakrabarty*, the Court altered the argument from a positive reason to limit the scope of patent rights to a narrow exclusion from the general rule of patentability. The phenomena of nature argument, after *Chakrabarty*, no longer stood on a moral foundation. Instead, it furthered the economic goal of encouraging inventive activity by distinguishing between abstract inventions that best promote such activity by remaining in the public domain and concrete inventions that best foster such activity by being subject to patent rights.

A second argument the *Chakrabarty* Court addressed further illustrates the close link between the market price of an invention and its patentability. Some of those opposed to Chakrabarty's patent claims argued that the grant of patent rights in genetically engineered organisms could have devastating social, health, and environmental consequences.[56] They argued that the Court should not agree to Chakrabarty's claim without first examining the effects that granting such rights would have on human health, the environment, and respect for life. They argued that such an examination would lead the Court to reject Chakrabarty's claim. That is, those opposed to Chakrabarty's claims argued that, to uphold the values of human dignity, human health, and environmental concern, the claims ought to be rejected.

The Court met this request to consider noneconomic values with a two-pronged response. First, the Court held that the noneconomic effects of granting a patent right to Chakrabarty would be minimal.[57] While the failure to gain patent rights in genetically engineered organisms might slow down the pace of research in this field,[58] no judicial decision, the Court held, would "deter the scientific mind from probing into the unknown any more than Canute could command the tides."

Second, the Court held that it was not competent to consider any but economic factors inhering in genetically engineered organisms.[59] Other ways of valuing such organisms—for example, in terms of their effect on health, the environment, and human dignity—were matters of "high policy" that only Congress could address. Congress, if it wished, could exempt genetically engineered organisms from the scope of patent law. Because Congress had not done so and because Congress had employed broad language to describe patentable subject matter, the Court stated that it had no choice but to accord a patent to Chakrabarty.

While the Court's response to the request to consider noneconomic factors begs many interesting questions,[60] I will pursue only one here. The Court failed to explain why evaluating the likely health, environmental, and dignity effects of granting a patent is any more speculative than determining the economic effects of such a grant. If, as the received learning informs us, the label "property" is granted to "encourage conduct we consider desirable" and is withheld "to discourage undesirable conduct," then why are health, the environment, and respect for life not included in the calculus of determining whether genetic research is conduct we consider desirable?[61] If examining the implications of patent rights on health, the environment, and dignity "involves the balancing of competing values and interests, which in our democratic system is the business of the elected representatives,"[62] then how could the Court have felt competent to address economic questions that touch on virtually all of these considerations?[63] If "the contentions now pressed" on the Court by those opposed to patenting genetically engineered organisms "should be addressed to the political branches of the Government, the Congress and the Executive, and not to the courts,"[64] then why should those in favor of patenting such organisms be able to address their contentions to the courts?

The *Chakrabarty* Court's myopic focus on economic value prevented it from asking how the grant of patent rights in genetically engineered organisms might affect the values of health, environmental responsibility, and respect for life. The phenomena of nature argument, in its previous incarnation in *Funk Brothers*, had treated inventions that threatened values similar to those ignored in *Chakrabarty* as unpatentable. By refocusing the phenomena of nature argument away from moral values toward economic value, the *Chakrabarty* Court closed off any discussion of the moral implications of its decision.

The cases examined in this chapter support the conclusion reached in chapter 3 that market price lies at the heart of property law. While the phenomena of nature argument opened the door to a discussion of noneconomic values inhering in inventions, the courts refused to step across the threshold and engage in such a discussion. As pointed out in chapter 3, courts prefer to base their property law decisions on economic value, believing that by ensuring a properly functioning market, they indirectly foster all values inhering in a good. In *Chakrabarty*, this attitude was taken to an extreme; when directly presented with serious noneconomic considerations, the Court concentrated exclusively on economics.

In the next chapter, I examine another series of cases, this time dealing with individuals' personae. Unlike most of the disputants in the cases examined in this chapter, those arguing for rights of control over their persona value this good not only in accordance with economic modes of valuation, but in accord with noneconomic modes as well. As will be discussed in the next chapter, even where the parties strongly value a disputed good in terms of noneconomic modes of valuation, the courts allocate rights to that good on the basis of economic modes of valuation. Like *Chakrabarty*, some of the cases examined in the next chapter illustrate the consequences of failing to directly consider noneconomic modes of valuation in allocating rights of control over goods. The principal of these is that not only do the courts ignore noneconomic modes of valuation in the allocation process, but the allocation process may itself actually undermine some of the ways in which we value disputed goods.

Chakrabarty illustrates how present-day courts might respond to Frankenstein's construction of his monster. As in *Chakrabarty*, Frankenstein created his creature out of existing biological material. The monster itself, like the bacterium in *Chakrabarty*, did not exist in nature. While *Funk Brothers* would have held that life is too inviolate to be patented, under *Chakrabarty* the courts could very well hold that Frankenstein had exercised ingenuity in creating something that had never existed and might, therefore, have accorded Frankenstein a patent in his monster. In response to those, like Frankenstein's fiancee and friends, who would argue that it degrades our humanity to patent life, that one must carefully consider the social and environmental effects of the grant of patent rights in living organisms, the courts would answer that they were not competent to deal with these questions. The exclusive concern of the courts would be to encourage invention. That they would have accomplished, but only by ignoring much.

5

Public Personae and Value

His fans snap up Elvis ashtrays, Elvis beach towels, Elvis on velvet and Elvis postage stamps. So why not Elvis glossy trading cards?

In October, Major League Marketing Inc., which sells Score and Pinnacle brand sports trading cards, will introduce a line of 660 Elvis Presley trading cards. The glossy pictures span the King's "Hound Dog" days as a gyrating teen idol to the twilight of his career as a Las Vegas showman.

Fans are already reaching for their wallets. Dan Shedrick, the company's president, said retail orders were double the company's original projections, though he would not disclose figures.[1]

Elvis the man may be dead, but his image, name, and persona live on. Posters and velvet paintings, decals and belt buckles, and films and television dramas point to the immortality of Elvis's public soul. This immortality did not arise through happenstance; it was carefully and consciously crafted through the efforts of Elvis and his manager, Colonel Tom Parker.[2] Elvis and Parker turned their creation of Elvis's public persona, with its attending adulation, into commercial gain by marketing merchandise bearing Elvis's name and likeness. They did so through the auspices of an independent corporation, the sole purpose of which was to handle the commercial exploitation of Elvis's persona. Even after Elvis died in 1977, Parker continued, through this corporation, to market Elvis merchandise and memorabilia.

Elvis was neither the first nor the last person to create a public persona. Countless entertainers, politicians, and even corporate heads have actively cultivated reputations among the public. Some have turned their reputation into political clout, others have relied on it to promote charitable causes,[3] and still others have translated their reputation into profit.[4] Further, just as the uses to which public figures have put their personae differ, so too did their motivations in creating these personae. Some aspired to fame for its own sake, while others cultivated celebrity in order to reach other goals such as respect, power, independence, philanthropy, or profit.

The complexity of motivations behind the creation of a public persona points to the fundamental difference between personae and the scientific discoveries and inventions examined in the previous chapter. One's persona, even if a public one and even if different from one's private self, is intimately connected with who one is. While the act of scientific discovery may be a source of pride or of identity, the thing discovered is removed from us. In contrast, not only is the act of creating a public persona linked to our identity—the choices we make in creating such a persona and our motivations for doing so tell much about who we are—but the thing created, the public persona, affects how others see us. The link between an individual and his or her persona is much stronger, therefore, than is the link between a scientist and his or her invention. Because of the strength of this link, the noneconomic values inhering in public personae are particularly forceful.

This chapter continues the inquiry into the link between property law and economic value by examining how courts resolve disputes centering on public personae. Given the close connection between these goods and values such as self-esteem, self-development, and human dignity, this examination tests the thesis stated in previous chapters that courts look only to a good's economic value in determining whether property rights ought to attach to that good. After reviewing cases dealing with the "right of publicity," the area of law protecting celebrities' commercial interests in their personae, this chapter concludes that this thesis applies despite the presence of significant noneconomic values inhering in such personae.

While supporting the thesis developed over the last few chapters, the analysis presented in this chapter will add some subtlety to it. The cases that I examine in this chapter illustrate that courts are not oblivious to the effects that their decisions may have on noneconomic modes of valuation. In fact, courts will occasionally stretch their analyses to find economic justifications for supporting the allocation of rights of control in order to vindicate noneconomic modes of valuation. But there are clear limits to the courts' willingness to stretch their analyses; there must be some plausible economic argument in favor

of awarding property rights even where the noneconomic values inhering in the disputed good appear overwhelming.

The subject matter of this chapter, public personae, possesses
interesting similarities with human biological materials. Both these
goods implicate values of identity, respect, and dignity. Both involve
one's body; in the case of personae, one's face and voice, and in the
case of human biological materials, physical components of the body.
We can therefore expect there to be parallels between the way the
courts have dealt with disputes concerning public personae and how
they would likely deal with a dispute concerning human biological
materials.

The cases this chapter examines arose when one individual used
the name, likeness, or persona of a public figure without that figure's
consent. Most often, the individual used the celebrity's name, likeness, or persona for commercial gain. That is, the individual attempted
to turn the celebrity's notoriety into a profit for her or himself. To
combat this unauthorized commercial use of their names, likenesses,
or personae by others, celebrities rely on their right of publicity.[5] This
right, the origins of which are found in the right of privacy—the right
to be left alone[6]—aims at protecting a celebrity's ability to control the
commercial use made of her or his persona.[7] The right of publicity
has several important characteristics. First, only public figures possess
it.[8] Other individuals must content themselves with the right of privacy, a right that endeavors to protect an individual's feelings rather
than the individual's commercial interests.[9] Second, under the right
of publicity, a celebrity is entitled to recover the wrongdoer's profits,
in addition to damages for hurt feelings.[10] Under the right of privacy,
by contrast, only the latter type of damages are available.[11] Third, the
predominant view is that the right of publicity survives the death of
the celebrity.[12] That is, the celebrity's estate and descendants continue
to have the exclusive right to exploit the celebrity's name, likeness,
and persona for commercial purposes after the celebrity has died.[13]
This again differs from the right of privacy, which does not survive
the right-holder's death.[14] Finally, the right of publicity is a personal
property right.[15] This legal conclusion, that the right of publicity is a
property right, is more or less the summation of the previous points;
when one has exclusive control over the right to sell or transfer and
the right to bequeath a good, it is not difficult to make the conclusion
that the good is one's personal property.

The right of publicity cases are particularly interesting in that
they provide a modern example of the creation and evolution of a

new property right.[16] Forty years ago, no such right existed. Then the courts created the right to sell the use of one's name and likeness. Over the course of the last forty years, the right has evolved into a fully assignable, descendible—that is, it is capable of being passed on to one's heirs at death—and exclusive right to the commercial value of one's name, likeness, voice, and identifying phrases. This evolution marked a change toward the economic valuation of celebrities' personae.

Crafting a Substitute Good

Like the property claimants surveyed in previous chapters, celebrities seeking to protect their personae have had to traverse two hurdles. These hurdles, identified in chapter 3, are that all parties to the dispute must value the contested good primarily in terms of its market price and that the award of property rights in the good must enhance, rather than hinder, trade in that good. If, in the cases examined in this chapter, the good in question had unambiguously been a public persona, one would likely find it difficult to negotiate these hurdles. This difficulty exists because the values inhering in public personae are immensely varied: for example, self-development, human dignity, self-worth, profit, and philanthropy. It is improbable that one motivation, the lure of the market value of one's persona, would predominate over the rest.[17]

The courts have, however, formulated an ingenious way to avoid the difficulty occasioned by the multitude of noneconomic values inhering in personae. Rather than grant a property right in the persona itself, courts grant such a right in a substitute good: the right of publicity. This right is the right to control the commercial use to which one's public persona is put.[18] While one may value one's persona in a variety of ways, one can only value the commercial use of that persona in terms of its economic value.[19] By thus crafting a new good to substitute for the celebrity's persona, courts ensure that all parties value the contested good in terms of its market price. This maneuver guarantees that the property claimant will successfully traverse the first hurdle.

While the substitution of a celebrity's persona with the right of publicity appears to leave certain aspects of the celebrity's persona out of the scope of the property right—namely, noncommercial values such as self-esteem and dignity—the courts have so expanded what is considered a commercial use of the celebrity's persona that little is, in practice, left unprotected. The solution of substituting one good, the right of publicity, for another, the celebrity's public persona, therefore has the salutary effect of ensuring that the property claimant will negotiate the first hurdle without reducing the scope of that claimant's property right.

This willingness to substitute one good for another solely to ensure property protection for a celebrity's persona illustrates the courts' desire to encourage the creation of such personae. While courts often leave the reasons for this desire unexpressed, they occasionally voice them. These reasons turn out to be the same as those that motivated courts to uphold or award property rights in *Moore v. Regents of the University of California* (to Dr. Golde),[20] *International News Service v. Associated Press*,[21] and *Diamond v. Chakrabarty*:[22] to encourage "the production of works of benefit to the public"[23] and to defend "the right of the individual to reap the reward of his endeavors."[24] Both of these concerns betray, as they did with respect to human biological materials, to news, and to living organisms, an economic motive for the courts' decision to award property rights in the form of the right of publicity.

The conclusion that the creation of personae is valuable to society, and thus worth encouraging through the allocation of property rights, tells little about how this determination of value was made. Courts do not state, for example, whether this determination is based on a conviction that personae are valuable in terms of self-development, that personae have an entertainment value, that personae are valuable because they boost the self-esteem of those who create them, or whether their value derives from the fact that someone is willing to pay for their use.[25] Many goods are valuable—friendship, happiness, and self-esteem, to name a few—without being property. Therefore, when a court holds that a good ought to be treated as property because it is valuable, one must take the court to be using the word "valuable" in a particular sense.

When courts declare that personae are valuable, they mean that personae have a market price.[26] Consider, for example, the language courts use in discussing the value of a celebrity's persona. Uniformly, courts highlight the commercial value of that persona.[27] While occasionally noting that the right of publicity, in addition to protecting a persona's commercial value, fosters such noneconomic values as respect,[28] self-esteem, and privacy,[29] courts do so only in passing.[30]

In most cases, however, courts make no attempt to identify a noneconomic value that is furthered through the award of the right of publicity; they are satisfied once they are convinced that a celebrity's persona is economically valuable.

Sowing and Reaping: a Reprise

The argument that a celebrity ought to be able "to reap the reward of his endeavors"[31] is a reprise of the sowing and reaping argument introduced in *International News Service v. Associated Press*.[32] It is no more compelling in the context of the right of publicity than it was in the context of the right to own news. To recapitulate, the sowing and reaping argument states that one ought to own what one has created through one's efforts. In the context of the right of publicity, the argument is that because celebrities have invested thought, skill, and labor in the creation of their public personae, they are entitled to the economic returns stemming from these personae.[33] The force of the argument derives from the form in which it is stated: as a moral proposition. This moral form merely camouflages, however, an economic calculation. As discussed in chapter 3,[34] the sowing and reaping argument, despite its moral facade, is no more than the economic conclusion that the award of property rights furthers trade in the good in question.

The creation of the right of publicity is premised on the belief that the award of such a right encourages the production of public personae that will, in turn, be traded on an open market. That is, courts believe that the grant of the right of publicity enhances trade in personae, thus satisfying the second hurdle to the award of property rights. While using the language of sowing and reaping, courts understand that the fundamental reason why they ought to create the right of publicity is that such a right provides a significant economic incentive to celebrities to create public personae.[35]

In its decision in *Zacchini v. Scripps-Howard Broadcasting Co.*,[36] the United States Supreme Court explained how the right of publicity fosters trade in personae. *Zacchini* arose because a television station, as part of its regular news program, broadcast the entire human cannonball performance of Zacchini at a county fair. Zacchini made his livelihood through these performances. When he noticed one of the station's reporters at his show, he requested that the station neither record nor broadcast his performance. The television station neverthe-less decided that the performance was news and broadcast it notwith-standing this request. In broadcasting Zacchini's performance, how-ever, the newscaster encouraged audience members to attend the fair to witness it in person. Zacchini sought damages against the television station for misappropriating his performance.

While the principal issue before the Court in *Zacchini* was whether the "right of publicity" interfered with the television station's right of free speech under the United States Constitution,[37] the Court discussed, at some length, the purpose of the right of publicity. This purpose was to encourage the production and dissemination of enter-tainment. The Court concluded that individuals require an economic incentive to create and disseminate entertainment.[38] In other words, according to the Court, individuals value public personae in market terms. By fostering market value, the Court held, the law can secure the production of entertaining performances. Individuals will create such performances as long as they receive an economic return. They will receive such a return so long as people are willing to pay for the performances. If the performances are entertaining, foster self-development, or are educational, people will be willing to pay for them. Therefore, although there are manifold values inhering in public personae, many of which are noneconomic, courts need concern them-selves only with market value.[39] The market can be relied upon to ensure that this market value reflects all the other values inhering in such personae.

The *Zacchini* Court held that the television station's broadcast of Zacchini's entire performance posed a serious threat to the economic value of the performance.[40] Since the public was freely given what it would normally have had to pay to see, Zacchini would not receive the economic rewards commensurate with the value—to the public, both economic and noneconomic—of his performance. Because of this, the market failed to translate this value into an economic incentive that would have encouraged Zacchini to create more performances.

The Court's discussion of the possibility that, rather than damp-ening attendance, the television broadcast may have actually increased attendance at Zacchini's live performance further illustrates the Court's exclusive concentration on economic value. The Court held that, should the broadcast have increased attendance, Zacchini would not have suffered any injury.[41] That is, the sole criterion in determining whether Zacchini was injured by the broadcast of his performance was whether he was economically injured. If Zacchini had other reasons why the broadcast bothered him—the lack of respect the television station demonstrated in refusing to accept his request not to film his performance, an antipathy toward television because it threatened live performance, the frivolity with which the station presented his performance, the manner in which the station broadcast the performance, that is, without the usual build-up of suspense—he could not recover unless he could prove economic injury. Therefore, to the Court, in the context of the right of publicity, values such as respect and integrity had no currency.

Creating a Descendible Right of Publicity

Since the 1950s, courts have held the right of publicity to be transferable. Subsequently, the right has evolved into a fully descendible one as well.[42] This evolution was prompted by the courts' desire to enable trade in public personae.[43] Since commercial interests in a persona, whether held by a purchaser or an heir, continue to exist after the death of a celebrity, there was no reason, courts held, that the right of publicity should die with the celebrity.[44] In fact, descendibility of the right of publicity furthered these commercial interests by stabilizing the market value of the right. Purchasers could buy the right to use a celebrity's persona without fear that this right would suddenly terminate should the celebrity unexpectedly die.[45] Those selling personae could receive the full commercial value of the personae without having to accept a discount against the possibility of an early death.[46] In sum, descendibility of the right of publicity removed some of the uncertainty relating to the market value of this right.

Courts had to overcome two obstacles in holding that the right of publicity fully survived the death of its creator. The first of these obstacles was the contention that the right of publicity was purely a personal right and, as such, could not survive the death of its creator. Those advancing this contention disputed the characterization of the right as being proprietary in nature. They argued that the right to control the commercial use of one's public persona was a species of the right of privacy, vindicating simply the personal right to be left alone. At bottom, this contention was premised on rejecting the application of economic norms to personae.

The opinion in *Memphis Development Foundation v. Factors Etc., Inc.*[47] exemplifies this rejection of the belief that one's public persona is merely an economic good. *Memphis Development* was one of several cases dealing with the right to exploit Elvis Presley's name and likeness after his death in 1977. While Presley was still alive, he had licensed Boxcar Enterprises to market merchandise bearing his name and likeness. Following Presley's death, Boxcar granted an exclusive sublicense to commercially exploit Presley's name and likeness to Factors Etc., Inc. Factors soon found itself fighting to protect this sublicense.

Memphis Development was a nonprofit corporation that solicited public contributions for the purpose of erecting a bronze statue of Presley in downtown Memphis. Donors who contributed $25 or more received an eight-inch pewter replica of the proposed statue. The foundation sought a declaratory judgment that Factors's license did not preclude the foundation's distribution of the replica statues. Factors counterclaimed, seeking an injunction to restrain the foundation from further distribution of the replicas.

The United States Court of Appeals for the Sixth Circuit took a noneconomic stance toward the question of whether the right of publicity survives the death of its creator. The court, purporting to apply Tennessee law, recognized that celebrities, while alive, have the exclusive right to the commercial use of their names and likenesses.[48] It rejected, however, Factors' contention that this right survived a celebrity's death. In doing so, the court adopted a very noneconomic characterization of the interests at stake. Instead of accepting the proposition that individuals create only when induced to do so by a financial incentive, the court undertook the task of identifying what motivates people to create public persona. The court argued that individuals create personae in order to achieve success and excellence, or because of a desire to contribute to or improve society, or for the emotional and financial rewards of achievement. Thus, while not discounting the incentive effect of financial compensation, the court held that this effect did not fully explain why individuals create public personae.

With this understanding of the motivations driving individuals to create personae, the *Memphis Development* court inquired into the effect that descendibility of the right of publicity would likely have on these motivations. The court examined both moral and economic effects. On the moral front, the court held that descendibility would only lead to the commercialization of the memory of one's predecessors. While children, for generations, have been content to receive their parents' good name, descendibility of the right of publicity would induce children of celebrities to view their parents as primarily a commodity with which to make a profit.[49] Thus, one of the motivations leading individuals to create personae, the desire to leave a good name to one's children, loses its force once that name is commercialized. The moral obligation to leave a good name becomes simply a financial one.

Despite its concern over noneconomic motivations, the court in *Memphis Development* devoted most of its time to analyzing the economic effects of recognizing a descendible right of publicity. Factors had argued that descendibility of the right of publicity encouraged individuals to create personae. The court dismissed this argument, contending that descendibility of the right of publicity provides only a weak incentive to create. Compared to such strong motivations as the desire to succeed or the desire to do good, the court held, the desire to ensure that one's heirs profit from one's persona is a weak motivation. Since descendibility of the right of publicity would provide no more than a weak incentive to create, the court concluded, descendibility was not necessary to induce creative effort.[50]

The *Memphis Development* court also relied on the anticompetitive effects of granting a descendible property right in one's persona. The court held that the grant of such a right would establish a stifling monopoly. Stating that the reason why the law provides monopolies in other areas such as patent law is to increase creative effort, the court concluded that descendibility of the right of publicity has no significant positive effect in motivating individuals to create personae. Descendibility merely provides a celebrity's heirs with a financial incentive to exploit that celebrity's likeness. There is no reason to expect, however, that these heirs will have any special expertise in exploiting their predecessor's persona. Thus, extending monopoly control over the celebrity's persona to that celebrity's heirs is unlikely to increase creative effort. Under these circumstances, the court concluded, it was best to leave the exploitation of the commercial value of a celebrity's persona to the market. If the celebrity's persona were available to all, those individuals with the necessary skill and know-how would be prompted to turn the persona into products available to all. Thus free trade, rather than a monopoly, best ensures creativity.

Reevaluating Descendibility: The Economic Argument

The *Memphis Development* court's voice was a lone one, however. Other courts wholeheartedly endorsed the view that the right of publicity survives its creator's death. In *Factors Etc. Inc. v. Pro Arts, Inc.*,[51] Pro Arts decided to market a poster of Presley within days of the latter's death. When Factors warned Pro Arts to discontinue marketing the poster, Pro Arts sought a declaratory judgment of noninfringement of any rights claimed by Factors. Factors responded by seeking an injunction to restrain Pro Arts from marketing the poster. This injunction was granted at trial. Pro Arts appealed to the United States Court of Appeals for the Second Circuit.

The central issue before the *Pro Arts* court was whether the right of publicity survived Presley's death. In contrast to the court in *Memphis Development*, the *Pro Arts* court took a purely economic view of this issue. The court noted that Presley had, during his life, validly transferred his right of publicity to Boxcar.[52] In doing so, he created for himself the right to receive a certain percentage of royalties from Boxcar. In other words, Presley had exchanged one property right, his right of publicity, for another right, the right to receive royalty payments. This transaction was a purely commercial one. Furthermore, Presley's death in no way altered the commercial viability of the transaction. The only change arising from Presley's death was that Presley's estate, rather than Presley himself, was entitled to the royalty payments. The market value of Presley's persona was in no way reduced by his death. Given this commercial reality, there was no reason not to recognize Boxcar's, and through Boxcar, Factors's, right to commercially exploit Presley's persona.

Not only was there no reason not to recognize the descendibility of Presley's right of publicity but, the *Pro Arts* court held, there was good reason to recognize its descendibility. In addition to Presley, both Boxcar and Factors had invested—financially—in the creation of Presley's persona. If the right of publicity did not survive Presley's death, then Boxcar and Factors would not be rewarded for their effort. Instead some third party, such as Pro Arts, would be able to swoop in and reap for itself the commercial value of Presley's persona, a commercial value that others had invested to create.

In yet another case dealing with Presley, *Tennessee ex rel. Elvis Presley International Memorial Foundation v. Crowell*,[53] the court also concluded that the right of publicity survived Presley's death. This holding effectively overruled *Memphis Development*.[54] In *Crowell*, a group of Presley fans organized the Elvis Presley International Foundation ("International Foundation") to raise money for a local hospital.

This foundation was incorporated in the state of Tennessee. Soon after, Presley's estate incorporated the Elvis Presley Memorial Foundation ("Memorial Foundation") to solicit money to build a fountain in a shopping center. In response to the Memorial Foundation's activities, the International Foundation commenced an action seeking to dissolve the Memorial Foundation. After losing at trial, the International Foundation appealed to the Tennessee Court of Appeals.

As in *Memphis Development* and in *Pro Arts*, the principal issue before the *Crowell* court was whether Presley's right of publicity survived him. The court rejected what it considered to be the *Memphis Development* court's "bias" against recognizing that the right of publicity is descendible.[55] Like the court in *Pro Arts*, the *Crowell* court viewed the right of publicity as a purely commercial good. Adopting this view, the *Crowell* court marshalled two broad economic arguments in support of its position that Presley's right of publicity survived him.[56] First, the court argued that the financial incentive provided by the descendibility of the right of publicity propelled individuals to invest time and effort into the development of their personae.[57] The *Crowell* court thus ignored the *Memphis Development* court's view that individuals are motivated by many factors in constructing a public persona; or, more precisely, the *Crowell* court ignored motivations other than money or goals translatable into money for spending time and effort in building a persona.

The second argument put forward by the court in *Crowell* was that descendibility is essential to protect the financial interests of those who invest in a celebrity's persona. Individuals will be less eager to invest in a celebrity's persona when there is uncertainty as to the length of time during which they will have to recoup on their investment.[58] Recognizing the right of publicity to be descendible removes this uncertainty, thus encouraging investment. Given that descendibility encourages both celebrities and investors to invest in the creation of public personae, the court concluded that the right of publicity ought to be descendible.

The evolution of the right of publicity toward descendibility began once the courts abandoned the view that many values inhere in a celebrity's persona in favor of the view that personae are commercial goods with a value determined by the market. Early concern over the morality of commercializing one's name gave way to concern over how best to commercialize that name. In parallel with this movement, the courts increasingly viewed the right of publicity as something different from the right of privacy; the former became a property right while the later remained a personal right.

Encouraging Exploitation during a Celebrity's Life

The second obstacle courts faced when considering whether the right of publicity ought to be fully descendible was the argument that descendibility ought only to be recognized if celebrities make use of the commercial value of their personae during their lives. This argument was forcefully stated in *Lugosi v. Universal Pictures*.[59] In that case Universal Pictures, for whom Bela Lugosi had performed in the movie *Dracula*, marketed Lugosi's image as Dracula after his death. Neither Universal nor Lugosi had exploited Lugosi's likeness during Lugosi's lifetime. Lugosi's estate brought suit against Universal, seeking both an injunction to prevent future use of Lugosi's image and damages for misappropriation.

The majority in *Lugosi* held that there are two components to the right of publicity. The first is the right to be left alone. Being tied to the right of privacy and thus a personal right, this component of the right of publicity dies with the celebrity. The second component is the right of a celebrity to tie his or her persona to a business or product; this combination results in a property right that can survive the celebrity. That is, by commercializing their personae, celebrities can transform their personal right into a property right. If, for whatever reason, a celebrity fails to exploit the commercial value of his or her persona during his or her life, then the opportunity to do so passes to the public.

The majority only obliquely explained why one's persona only becomes property when one exploits its commercial value. One explanation for the link between property rights and commercial exploitation is an economic one: that by providing only those who exploit their personae with a property right, the court ensures that the creation of personae is maximized. Behind this explanation lies the following argument. The opportunity to develop a good into a marketable product ought to belong to those who are willing to invest time and effort in such development.[60] Since celebrities are in the best position to exploit their own personae, the law ought to provide them with a strong incentive to do so. Permitting a celebrity to sell the use of her or his persona in perpetuity offers that celebrity a greater financial incentive—through a higher purchase price—to invest in her or his persona than if the celebrity were only able to assign the use of the persona during her or his life.[61] If a celebrity does not, however, take advantage of the commercial value of her or his persona during her or his life, then the law ought to encourage others to do so. Since a celebrity's heir is no more likely than anyone else to exploit the celebrity's persona, the right to use that persona ought to be available to all.

The dissent in *Lugosi* also relied on economic arguments in analyzing the issue of whether the right of publicity ought to survive the death of a celebrity whether or not that celebrity exploited the commercial value of his or her persona during his or her life. The dissent held that descendibility encourages creative effort.[62] Individuals are more likely to invest in the creation of their personae when they know that they can transfer control over the use of their personae to a suitable beneficiary. Descendibility should not depend on whether the celebrity exploited his or her persona during life. An individual may not have exploited the commercial value of his or her persona while alive because the appropriate opportunity had not arisen or because he or she wished to pass on this opportunity to his or her heirs. Further, it would often be difficult to determine whether an individual had sufficiently exploited his or her personae while alive to warrant descendibility of the right of publicity. Not only would this difficulty introduce uncertainty, but it may lead to abuse of the unwary. The right of publicity should, the dissent therefore concluded, always be descendible.

Fitting the Round Peg of Respect into the Square Hole of Economics

Another case dealing with the issue of whether the right of publicity is descendible only if celebrities exploit the commercial value of their personae during their lives is *Martin Luther King, Jr., Center for Social Change, Inc. v. American Heritage Products, Inc.*[63] In *King*, American Heritage Products marketed a plastic bust of Martin Luther King, Jr. King's estate brought action to enjoin American Heritage from making this use of King's likeness. Because the issue of a right of publicity involved state law, the United States Court of Appeals for the Eleventh

Circuit certified certain questions to the Supreme Court of Georgia.[64] Judgment was entered in accordance with the supreme court's reasons.

The *King* court held that descendibility of the right of publicity serves an important purpose: it encourages the creation of public personae. Descendibility encourages such creation by increasing the market value of celebrities' personae during their lives, thereby providing celebrities with an additional financial incentive to invest in their personae.[65] Descendibility has this effect on a persona's market value because it ensures investors that their interest in a particular celebrity's persona is not contingent on that celebrity remaining alive. Investors, under these circumstances, are therefore willing to pay more for the persona than they would be if the right of publicity were not descendible. Thus, by protecting the economic value of a celebrity's persona even after death against those who have neither invested nor created, the law maximizes creative effort.

The *King* court's analysis suddenly veered off its economic course, however, when faced with the question of whether the right of publicity ought only to be descendible if its creator commercially exploited it during her or his lifetime. The court's entire opinion, until confronted by this question, centered on encouraging creation by offering celebrities the opportunity to exploit their personae.[66] However, when addressing the need for exploitation of a persona during its creator's lifetime, the court abruptly altered its focus. Rather than encourage the creation of personae, the court sought to protect respect for, and the memory of, King. The court's reversal of direction was complete; the court went as far as arguing that the right of publicity ought to be descendible without the celebrity having had to exploit her or his persona while alive because this provided less of an incentive to exploit one's persona. Thus, not only did the court abandon its offer of commercial exploitation as an incentive to create, but it viewed such exploitation as a hazard to be avoided.

The first part of the *King* opinion, in which the court aimed at promoting creation through the offer of commercial exploitation, lived side-by-side and in conflict with the last part of the opinion, in which the court aimed at avoiding commercial exploitation. In attempting to produce some harmony between these two parts, the court stated, in a footnote, that the goals of encouraging respect for and protecting the memory of public figures—the goals behind the decision that celebrities need not exploit their personae in order for the right of publicity to survive them—could also support the conclusion that the right of publicity ought to be descendible.[67] The court did not, however, go so far as to rewrite its reasons with respect to descendibility. The contradiction thus remained.

The *King* court recognized that many values inhere in public personae. The court understood that a person may invest in the creation of one's own persona without expectation or desire of profit.[68] Given this understanding, it is somewhat surprising that the court felt compelled to ground its recognition of the right of publicity in the need to offer commercial exploitation of personae as an incentive to create such personae. No court had a better opportunity than the one sitting in *King*, in which the facts overwhelmingly demonstrated the noneconomic reasons for King having achieved fame, to base the right of publicity on noneconomic values. That the *King* court declined this opportunity further illustrates the fundamental link that this and previous chapters have elucidated between economic value and property law.

Expanding the Scope of the Right of Publicity

Just as the rapid evolution of the right of publicity into a fully descendible right illustrates the courts' goal of fostering the economic value of a celebrity's persona, the expansion of the scope of that right, to include ever more aspects of a celebrity's personality, reveals the desire to increase the quantum of that value. Not only is a celebrity's name and likeness protected against commercial exploitation, but the law now recognizes a celebrity's right to the exclusive commercial use of her or his voice[69] and of phrases associated with the celebrity.[70] The simultaneity of the evolution toward expansion and the evolution toward descendibility is not a random occurrence; both are predicated on property law's central concern for economic value.

The debate over how wide a scope should be given to the right of publicity turned on the question of how to balance the powers of free trade and monopoly so as to maximize creative effort. Recall that this question also controlled the debate, examined in chapter 4, over whether computer programs and new organisms ought to be patentable. The argument against the grant of property protection is that such protection impedes creative effort by blocking access to public personae. Without this access, individuals will be deprived of the opportunity to use such personae in new and useful ways. Thus, less invention is likely to follow. The argument for expanding the scope of the right of publicity is that the greater the control one has over the use of one's own persona, the greater the incentive one has to commercially exploit it. That is, the more aspects of one's personality that one can sell, the greater the profit to be made from selling it.

The opinions of the majority and the dissent in *Carson v. Here's Johnny Portable Toilets*[71] illustrate the nature of the debate. In *Carson*, a manufacturer of portable toilets called itself "Here's Johnny Portable Toilets" in order to capitalize on the phrase "Here's Johnny," used to introduce Johnny Carson on the *Tonight Show* and elsewhere. The manufacturer coupled its name with another phrase, "The World's Foremost Commodian," to further play with the reference to Johnny Carson. Carson, who used his name to market a chain of restaurants and a line of clothing, brought suit against the toilet manufacturer, alleging a breach of his right of publicity. The trial court rejected Carson's claim, holding that Carson's right of publicity was limited to his name and likeness; it did not include the exclusive right to exploit phrases associated with him.

The United States Court of Appeals for the Sixth Circuit overturned the trial court ruling and held that the right of publicity is premised on protecting a celebrity's financial interest in the commercial exploitation of his or her "identity."[72] A celebrity's identity, the court stated, goes well beyond the celebrity's name and likeness; it includes anything that would identify the celebrity in the public eye. Every aspect of a celebrity's identity must be constructed through hard work. In order to induce celebrities, therefore, to undertake such work, the law must provide them with the economic incentive to do so. This incentive, the court argued, is provided by granting celebrities the exclusive right to commercially exploit all aspects of their personae, including phrases identified with such celebrities.

The dissent in *Carson* argued that granting a wide scope to the right of publicity prevents others from making creative use of phrases that may be associated with certain celebrities. That is, if the mere use of a phrase by a celebrity is sufficient to take that phrase out of the public domain, the stock of phrases available for future creative effort will be decreased.[73] While agreeing that the purpose of the right of publicity was to encourage individuals to invest in their personae, the dissent contended that extending this right to include phrases merely associated with a celebrity did not further this purpose. It is true, the dissent conceded, that individuals must put time, effort, and skill into creating a well-known name and likeness; however, it is not true that Carson expended any time, effort, or skill to associate the phrase "Here's Johnny" with himself. Therefore, the dissent argued, there is no need to provide celebrities with a financial incentive to associate such phrases with themselves.

Granting a monopoly right over a phrase merely associated with Carson, the *Carson* dissent continued, would have a negative economic impact. Carson would have taken away something from society, the right to use the phrase "Here's Johnny," without having contributed something to society in return.[74] Thus society suffers because the stock of phrases available to others has been reduced by one and society has received no compensating good in return. The dissent further held that expanding the scope of the right of publicity would have a chilling effect on commercial innovation and opportunity.[75] Individuals would be dissuaded from undertaking creative effort out of fear that they may unknowingly use a phrase that a celebrity had already associated with her or himself.[76]

The drive to expand the right of publicity to cover all identifying characteristics of a celebrity stemmed from a purely economic appreciation of public personae. Other values inhering in such personae were ignored in the courts' efforts to foster and enhance the market value of personae. Consider again, for example, the United States Supreme Court decision in *Zacchini v. Scripps-Howard Broadcasting Co.*[77] In affirming the right of publicity, the Court held that a television station had no right under the First Amendment to broadcast, as part of its news broadcast, Zacchini's performance. In effect, Zacchini's right of publicity in his performance trumped the station's free speech right to broadcast that performance. Given the ferocity with which courts usually defend free speech values,[78] the Court's choice to vindicate the economic value of Zacchini's performance is a strong portent that, given a choice between an economic value and any other value, courts will choose the former.[79]

Reintegrating the Right of Privacy

Once the courts had securely fixed the right of publicity to a commercial foundation and gone to the trouble of detaching this right from the right of privacy, they nonetheless began the process of reintegrating the right of privacy into the right of publicity. This reintegration occurred, however, by subordinating the right of privacy to the right of publicity. That is, courts transformed the right of privacy into a right that, if not actually premised on the promotion of economic values, had the effect of furthering them.

The case of *Waits v. Frito-Lay, Inc.*[80] illustrates the attempt to reintroduce the right of privacy into the right of publicity. In *Waits*, Frito-Lay commissioned Tracy-Locke, Inc. to produce a radio commercial publicizing the introduction of a new snack food. Tracy-Locke seized upon the idea of using the sound and feel of Tom Waits's song, "Step Right Up."[81] Tracy-Locke searched for and found a singer who could imitate Waits's voice and style. Using this singer, Tracy-Locke produced a commercial with a song that, to members of the general public, sounded as if it had been sung by Waits.

Frito-Lay's imitation of his voice upset Waits because he had a policy against endorsing products. Moreover, this policy was a public one; Waits had often expressed his belief that artists who participate in making commercials jeopardize their artistic integrity. Thus, when friends and fans heard the Frito-Lay commercial, they were surprised to hear someone they believed was Waits endorsing a commercial product. Waits felt humiliated and brought suit. A jury found that Frito-Lay had violated Waits's right of publicity and awarded him damages not only for his economic but for his emotional injury as well. Frito-Lay appealed against this verdict and damage award to the United States Court of Appeals for the Ninth Circuit.

The *Waits* court rejected Frito-Lay's argument that the right of publicity did not include the right to control the commercial use of one's voice. In so doing, the court relied on an argument similar to that used by the majority in *Carson*. The court stated that Waits's voice was an identifying characteristic.[82] Agreeing with the *Carson* majority, the court held that celebrities have a right of publicity in all aspects of their identity. Thus, the court found that Waits had a property right in his voice.

Far more interesting, however, was the *Waits* court's determination that Waits was entitled to damages not only for his economic injury but for the injury to his feelings and to his reputation. This is interesting because it illustrates the reintroduction of the right of privacy into the right of publicity. This reintroduction occurs, however, only at the cost of putting commercial interests ahead of privacy interests.

The right of privacy, one may remember, serves to protect individuals from hurt feelings, such as embarrassment and humiliation. The right of publicity broke away from the right of privacy on this point, as it was aimed at vindicating a celebrity's commercial interests and had little to do with hurt feelings or damaged reputations.[83] The *Waits* court held, however, that Waits was entitled to damages for his feelings of humiliation following the broadcast of the Frito-Lay commercial.[84] Nor was the *Waits* court exceptional in thus holding; previous courts had come to the same conclusion.[85] The further finding that Waits could recover for injury to his reputation[86] was similarly in line with precedent.[87]

What the *Waits* case highlights is the degree to which a celebrity can recover, through the right of publicity, exactly what an individual can recover under the right of privacy. That is, a celebrity can use the right of publicity as a surrogate for the right of privacy. There is a catch, however. In order to recover privacy-like damages, a celebrity has to prove a violation of his or her commercial interests. Absent these interests, a celebrity has no right of publicity and no ability, using that right, to collect privacy damages. Celebrities' privacy interests are thus dependent on their commercial interests.

The *Waits* case embodies this subjugation of privacy to commercial concerns. As stated earlier, Waits had no desire to commercially exploit any aspect of his identity, including his voice. His only interest in suing Frito-Lay was to prevent it from further embarrassing him. In order to win his suit, however, and thus vindicate his privacy interest, Waits had to claim a violation of his commercial interests. That is, Waits had to claim that Frito-Lay had violated his financial interests in his voice. But, given Waits's attitude toward celebrity endorsement of products, he had no desire to commercially exploit his persona as embodied in his voice.[88] Waits had to maintain, therefore, a facade of commercial exploitation in order to vindicate his true interest: his integrity. If, however, Waits had not been able to claim a commercial interest in his voice—for example, if the courts had not expanded the scope of the right of publicity to include one's voice—he would not have been able to recover, under the right of publicity, for his embarrassment. *Waits* therefore teaches us once again that, when it comes to the right of publicity, the most important value inhering in one's persona is its market value. Other values will be vindicated, but only if their vindication is consistent with the vindication of the persona's economic value.

The law pertaining to the right of publicity has followed a clear course since its inception in the 1950s. Every development since the decision that the right of publicity is transferable, through the decision that it is descendible, to the determination that all identifying characteristics of a celebrity's identity are protected, has been motivated by the desire to foster and increase the market value of public personae. The courts have willingly subordinated other values inhering in such personae in order to fulfill this desire. This despite the strong noneconomic values inhering in personae such as self-development, self-esteem, respect, and dignity.

The presentation of property discourse presented in earlier chapters can be refined somewhat in light of the cases I have examined in this chapter. Although courts look to the encouragement of economic modes of valuation when allocating property rights, they are not oblivious to the possible salutary effects that this allocation may have on noneconomic modes of valuation. But despite this concern for noneconomic modes of valuation, the courts are unwilling to confer property rights where the only purpose for doing so is the vindication of a noneconomic mode of valuation; the courts must first find an economic reason to justify such a conferral of rights.

The acknowledgment that noneconomic modes of valuation are important have, however, clear limits. Courts are willing to strain economic reasoning only so far in order to accommodate noneconomic modes of valuation. In the next chapter I will study two cases in which those seeking rights did so in order to vindicate their noneconomic valuation of the good in dispute. In one case, the court found an economic basis to award the right while in the other, despite the obvious strength of the noneconomic values at stake, the court refused to award the right because it could find no economic basis on which to grant it.

6

Hiding behind Economic Values

> The [German] constitution was amended at the end of 1992 to limit the right of asylum. The number of asylum-seekers dropped from 438,200 in 1992 to 322,600 in 1993. It is running now at around 8,000 a month and would be even less but for refugees from the Yugoslav war.[1]

Germany has a very restrictive immigration law and, until 1993, had a very liberal refugee law.[2] Anyone who claimed to be a political refugee was virtually guaranteed of being permitted to live and work in Germany for at least several years. People who were interested in immigrating to Germany, but who could not meet the stringent requirements of the immigration laws, therefore claimed to be political refugees even though they had no legitimate claim to be such. When the number of people thus circumventing its immigration laws turned into a torrent, Germany changed its refugee law. It is now much more difficult to gain admittance into Germany as a refugee. In the result, there are still many people who wish to immigrate to Germany but who can find no way of doing so.

Like the immigrant who can only gain admittance by feigning to be a refugee, individuals who hope to vindicate their nonmarket interests in a good must pretend, in a property suit, that they value the good in terms of its market price or in a way that can be converted into a market price. Property law, as illustrated in the last three chapters, is directly attentive only to the market values of goods. Only if a good is a market good and if granting a property right in that good is likely to enhance trade in it will the courts award such rights. However many noneconomic values inhere in a good, property law does not directly seek to further them. This does not mean the courts are unmindful of these values; rather, courts leave the vindication of these values to market action. They do so on the following set of assumptions. Courts recognize that individuals value goods in many, occasionally contradictory, ways. Courts assume, however, that each individual places a monetary value upon his or her particular way of valuing the good. The person who values the good the most, the assumption continues, will attach the highest money price to it. In a free market in which goods are openly traded and in the absence of high transaction costs, the individual willing to pay the most for a good—by definition in economics, the person who values the good the most—will buy it. In this fashion, market forces direct the good to the individual who values it the most. Best of all, this allocation does not require the courts to weigh or to compare the values inhering in the good.

Courts adjudicating property claims thus seek to ensure that there is a functioning market in contested goods. By securing open access to such goods and by protecting the goods' market price from erosion due to uncertainty as to title, courts set the stage for market action. Directly concerning themselves with such noneconomic values as self-development, self-esteem, or human health serves no purpose, as such values do not directly count in the courts' economic arithmetic. In adjudicating property claims, therefore, courts assume that they can safely ignore such noneconomic values, no matter how substantial or pressing those values appear in the particular case. Thus, in *Diamond v. Chakrabarty*,[3] despite warnings concerning the environmental and health consequences of encouraging genetic research, the United States Supreme Court held these noneconomic concerns to be irrelevant to its property-law decision. In *Martin Luther King, Jr., Center for Social Change v. American Heritage Products*,[4] in spite of the estate's clear and exclusive concern for the memory of King, the court grounded its decision to award a property right on the basis of economic values. Even the court's last-minute conversion to noneconomic forms of valuation was half-hearted; it made no substantial attempt to ground the estate's property right in anything but economic value.

Of the property claimants surveyed in previous chapters, Tom Waits[5] most resembles the immigrant claiming refugee status. Waits had no interest in the market value of his persona; in fact, he publicly disclaimed any such interest. Nevertheless, because the law of property recognizes only market values, Waits had to claim injury to the market value of his voice in order to vindicate the noneconomic ways he did value his voice. Waits thus feigned an economic interest in order to defend his integrity. Waits was fortunate that he could sufficiently manipulate his claim so as to fit within property law's requirement that one be economically motivated. Not all those who value goods in nonmarket ways are so fortunate.

This chapter concludes the discussion begun in chapter 3 concerning the link between property law and market value. The three previous chapters have investigated how property law treats goods, ranging from purely market goods to highly personal goods, and have illustrated that only those claimants who can demonstrate an overriding interest in the market value of a good will receive property rights to the good. Courts treat goods in which significant nonmarket values such as health, self-esteem, and dignity inhere in no different fashion, except at the margins, than they treat purely commercial goods. Thus, courts grant property rights to personae, in which many nonmarket interests inhere, for the same reasons that they grant such rights to glorified radio commercials, which have only a market value.[6]

I have spent a significant amount of time examining the nature of property discourse as practiced in American courtrooms. The purpose of this examination has been to determine what would likely be the effect of applying this discourse to human biological materials. The effect will extend far beyond the courtroom, as the application of property discourse will result in the award of rights of control over these goods to certain individuals but not to others. To the extent that we, as a society, care about how and for which purposes human biological materials are put, we ought all to be concerned that these rights of control are allocated on a basis that fairly represents all the ways that we value these materials. As I have been arguing, our application of property discourse to human biological materials is likely to result in an allocation of rights on a basis that ignores some of the most fundamental ways that we value human biological materials.

This chapter rounds out the analysis undertaken thus far by examining two cases in which the property claimants were centrally concerned with noneconomic values inhering in the contested good. In the first of these cases, the property claimant fitted its noneconomic way of valuing the contested good with a market facade. This claimant won a property right and used it to prevent harm to its noneconomic interests. In the second case, the claimants were not so successful. Although they convinced the courts hearing their case of the vital importance of their noneconomic interests in the contested good, they could not frame their way of valuing the good in terms of economic value. They thus lost their case.

The analysis of the two cases that I undertake in this chapter completes the argument, made throughout the preceding three chapters, that if human biological materials are to be treated as property, they will be valued primarily in terms of their market price. Decisions as to who ought to own such materials, to what uses these materials ought to be put, and who should benefit from their use will all be formulated within a context that esteems economic values above all others. The implications of making such decisions on market principles will be left for consideration until the next chapters. The aim of this chapter is, however, to establish that the law will value human biological materials in terms of market price.

Artistic Integrity

In *Gilliam v. American Broadcasting Co.,*[7] Monty Python, the British comedy troupe, sought to enjoin ABC from broadcasting a television program consisting of significantly edited and rearranged comedy shows written and performed by the troupe. The shows had originally aired in England, under the name "Monty Python's Flying Circus," pursuant to a scriptwriters' agreement between Monty Python and the British Broadcasting Company. Under the agreement, the BBC could not alter scripts submitted by Monty Python, except in minor ways, unless it first consulted with the comedy troupe. The BBC also had the authority to license the broadcast of the shows outside of England. Apart from this authority to alter scripts prior to production of the actual episodes and to license foreign broadcasts of the show, the BBC retained no rights to the scripts.

Although noncommercial and some small commercial American broadcasters had aired several "Monty Python's Flying Circus" shows, the first large commercial broadcaster to become interested in these shows was ABC. ABC hoped to broadcast excerpts from various "Monty Python's Flying Circus" episodes. It therefore approached the comedy troupe seeking rights to such a broadcast but was rebuffed because Monty Python believed the proposed format to be too disjointed. Meanwhile, Time-Life Films acquired the rights to the shows from the BBC. In its agreement with the BBC, Time-Life was given the right to edit the shows in order to insert commercials and to censor objectionable material. (The scriptwriters' agreement between Monty Python and the BBC had provided no such right.) Time-Life then licensed ABC to broadcast the shows.

ABC proposed to broadcast a total of six half-hour "Monty Python's Flying Circus" shows in two 90-minute specials. Given that, out of every 90 minutes of broadcast time, 24 minutes are normally devoted to commercials, Monty Python members feared that the shows would be severely edited. BBC officials promised that the shows would be broadcast back-to-back in their entirety. The troupe accepted this assurance. When ABC broadcast the first of the two specials in early October 1975, members of Monty Python angrily discovered that ABC had heavily edited the shows in order to fit in commercials and to remove objectionable material. The comedy troupe felt that its shows had been mutilated.

When Monty Python later learned that ABC intended to broadcast a second special in December, it approached ABC to negotiate a delay. These negotiations failed. Monty Python then commenced an action to prevent ABC's broadcast of the second special and any rebroadcast of the first special. After instituting its action, Monty Python sought a preliminary injunction to enjoin ABC from airing the second special. The troupe argued that by altering the sequence of the original shows, ABC had misappropriated the underlying scripts. These scripts, Monty Python contended, belonged to the troupe. The trial court sympathized with Monty Python's predicament, holding that ABC had severely distorted the original "Monty Python's Flying Circus" shows. The judge held, however, that Monty Python had not established its ownership of the underlying scripts. The judge also found that ABC would be irreparably harmed if it could not broadcast the second special. He therefore refused to grant the requested injunction. Monty Python appealed against this ruling. By the time the appeal was heard, however, ABC had broadcast the second special. Monty Python thus sought a preliminary injunction to prevent any future broadcasts of the two specials. The United States Court of Appeals for the Second Circuit granted this relief.

I have set out the facts in *Gilliam* in some detail in order to highlight Monty Python's consistent concern over the presentation of its work. In its scriptwriters' agreement with the BBC, in its rejection of ABC's initial offer to broadcast segments of "Monty Python's Flying Circus" shows, in its concern that ABC might edit the shows in order to fit three commercial-free 30-minute shows into a 90-minute special with commercials, and in seeking an injunction to prevent the broadcast of the edited shows, the comedy troupe demonstrated a keen interest in maintaining the artistic integrity of its work. While Monty Python could have compromised this integrity in order to capture greater profits—it could, for example, have agreed to ABC's first proposal to air the shows in edited form—the troupe decided not to do so.

Gilliam provides, as the preceding discussion suggests, an example of a party seeking to use property law in order to vindicate noneconomic values. Like Tom Waits, Monty Python claimed an infringement of a property right in order to preserve the noneconomic way in which it valued its artistic integrity. Instead, however, of relying on this noneconomic interest to support its property claim, Monty Python presented its case to the United States Court of Appeals for the Second Circuit as one involving primarily economic values. By repackaging its case as one implicating economic values, Monty Python provided the court with a peg on which to hang its decision to award a property right to the troupe. Absent such a peg, Monty Python would likely have been unable to vindicate its artistic integrity.

Monty Python claimed a common-law copyright in its script. The BBC's right to the recorded television shows did not displace this copyright, Monty Python maintained, because the shows were derivative of the script. Copyright protection of derivative works, the troupe contended, is limited to additions made to the derivative work over what existed in the underlying work. Therefore, according to Monty Python, the BBC had no legal authority to permit Time-Life to edit the "Monty Python's Flying Circus" shows.

The Court of Appeals for the Second Circuit agreed that Monty Python retained its copyright in its scripts and that the agreement between the BBC and Time-Life did not derogate from this right.[8] The court found that ABC infringed this copyright by editing the recorded shows without having first consulted with Monty Python. Copyright law is premised, the court stated, on encouraging the production of artistic work by providing adequate market protection to the creators of such work. ABC's broadcast threatened Monty Python's market interest in its shows. By distorting the nature of the comedy troupe's work through heavy editing, ABC presented Monty Python to its first nationwide American audience in an unflattering light. Many members of the audience, having never before experienced the comedy of Monty Python, would have believed that the ABC broadcasts fairly represented the troupe's brand of comedy. Many such members would thus be disinclined to patronize the work of Monty Python in the future. This would injure the troupe financially.

Monty Python did not rest its claim to an injunction on its market argument alone; the troupe also maintained that the court should

grant the injunction on the basis of its artistic rights. The troupe
argued that it had the right not to have its art deformed by others.[9]
ABC had done precisely this when it broadcast mutilated versions of
"Monty Python's Flying Circus." In so doing, ABC compromised
Monty Python's nonmarket interest in the artistic integrity of its work.
For this violation, the troupe concluded, ABC ought to be held liable.

The court of appeals agreed with Monty Python that ABC had
undermined the artistic integrity of the troupe's work by broadcasting
the troupe's shows in an edited form. The court also agreed that ABC
should be held liable for subverting Monty Python's artistic integrity.
The theory upon which the court based this conclusion differed significantly, however, from that proposed by Monty Python. The court's
theory was firmly rooted in economic analysis.

Monty Python's motivation for seeking the injunction against
ABC was, as discussed earlier, to protect the troupe's artistic integrity.
Monty Python's commercial interests were secondary at best. Consider the economic reality of the case. Monty Python had never before
received national exposure in the United States. ABC's broadcasts of
the troupe's edited shows, even if of a lower quality than the unedited
versions, brought Monty Python's humor to millions who would not
otherwise have heard of the troupe. Even if the majority of the audience cared never again to watch a Monty Python performance, this
still left thousands, if not hundreds of thousands, who would keep
an open mind with respect to the troupe. This large new audience
meant additional money to the troupe by way of future sales. Thus,
even though its shows were mutilated, and even though it might
have attracted a larger audience had they not been edited, Monty
Python was well ahead, financially, of the position it would have been
in had ABC not broadcast any show. In addition, Monty Python could
not realistically hope, given the realities of network broadcasting, to
have its shows aired without significant editing for commercials. No
major network would broadcast the troupe's work unless it was made
to conform to American television standards of eight minutes of commercials for each half-hour period. Therefore, if Monty Python had
been truly concerned about maximizing its economic well-being, it
would have approved of ABC's broadcasts and, in fact, would have
agreed to the earlier request to broadcast excerpts from "Monty Python's Flying Circus."

The Court of Appeals for the Second Circuit upheld Monty Python's right to the artistic integrity of its work not out of a desire to
directly further artistic integrity but on the basis of protecting Monty

Python's market interests in its shows. Artists such as the Monty Python troupe, the court argued, have a market interest in pleasing their audience. The more audience members enjoy the artists' work, the more willing they will be to pay for such enjoyment and the larger the audience will become. Therefore artists create their work, according to this argument, in order to suit the tastes of their audience. Artists who cannot make their work conform to the tastes of their audience will suffer financially and, eventually, will be driven out of the art market. In this way the market encourages those artists with skill and insight capable of rousing the public imagination to continue with their work and encourages the rest to change careers.

Should a third party present the public with a distorted version of an artist's work, the court's argument continued, that third party would threaten the economic well-being of the artist. This is so because the distortion, if significant, undermines the artist's effort to create work that pleases her or his audience. Being less pleased, the artist's audience will pay less for the artist's work. The artist will thus suffer financially and will produce less work. Such a result is economically inefficient; society will be deprived of pleasing artwork. Therefore, in order to encourage the production of quality artwork, the law ought to recognize an artist's right to the artistic integrity of her or his work.[10]

The court of appeals was not oblivious to the salutary consequences that its economic analysis had on the vindication of the value of artistic integrity. In fact, it is possible that the court was motivated to construct its economic argument in order to be able to vindicate this value. This possibility can be inferred from the fact that the court's economic argument was strained at best. After all, the creation of artwork is dissimilar from the creation of widgets. Much of what is presently considered "good" art was, at the time of its creation, considered poor by the art market.[11] This is because talented artists often lead, rather than follow, public taste. Thus, there is not necessarily a correlation between a work's price on the market and its artistic value. Similarly, the idea of tampering does not apply to artwork in the same way that it applies to cars or drugs. The distortion of a piece of art may not lessen its value, and, in some circumstances, may actually add value—aesthetically.[12]

The court of appeals's decision to found Monty Python's property right in its script on an inapposite economic analogy between artwork and manufactured goods rather than on the value of artistic integrity calls for an explanation. I suggest that the most cogent explanation is that property rights are founded on economic value. Courts award property rights to a good when to do so enhances trade in that good. Thus courts, from *International News Service v. Associated Press*[13] through the Court in *Diamond v. Chakrabarty*[14] to *Zacchini v. Scripps-Howard Broadcasting Co.*,[15] upheld the allocation of property rights to goods that had not theretofore been subject to property law on the basis of promoting trade in those goods. Even where the courts' motivation for the accord of property rights was noneconomic, as in *Martin Luther King, Jr., Center for Social Change v. American Heritage Products, Inc.*,[16] *Waits v. Frito-Lay, Inc.*,[17] and *Gilliam*, they nevertheless justified their decision to award such rights on the basis of promoting trade. While the courts in the latter cases pushed and twisted economic analysis to arrive at the desired result, they did not push too far. The courts consistently advanced at least plausible, if not ultimately convincing, economic arguments in support of the award of property rights.

Gilliam illustrates how parties wishing to vindicate some noneconomic values inhering in a good can manipulate property-law discourse, premised on purely economic considerations, to achieve their ends. While these parties, and the courts they try to convince, must operate within the confines of the goal of promoting trade, they can often persuasively argue that granting them property rights achieves this goal. Sometimes parties make such arguments with a wink and a nod, knowing full well that they are highly contrived. Other times, they actually believe their economic contentions. Nevertheless, parties do not, where possible, directly found their property claims on noneconomic values. To the extent that they rely on these values at all, they do so only in a secondary way.

Protection of a Community

Local 1330, United Steel Workers of America v. United States Steel Corp.[18] provides an example of a party that, in attempting to vindicate the noneconomic value of community, could make no plausible economic argument in favor of its claimed property right. The case involves the decision by U.S. Steel to shut down two steel mills in Youngstown, Ohio. The company's stated reason for shutting the plants down was that they were obsolete and thus unprofitable.

The community of Youngstown was built around steel and, in particular, around U.S. Steel. Because of steel there were jobs, there were schools, there were roads, and there was expansion.[19] The fate of the community was intimately tied to the future of U.S. Steel's two mills. Given this situation, the company's decision to leave Youngstown was likely to completely devastate the community.

In order to avoid the devastation of their community, the local steelworkers' union, the local congressman, and the Attorney General of Ohio commenced an action against U.S. Steel in an attempt to force the company to keep the two mills operational and, in the alternative, to sell the mills to the community. U.S. Steel claimed that it had the absolute right to make the business decision to shut down the plants. When the union sought to negotiate for the purchase of the mills, U.S. Steel refused, claiming that it feared the government would subsidize the operation of the mills to the competitive detriment of the company.[20]

The trial court was initially extremely sympathetic to the union's claim. At a pretrial hearing, the district judge stated his fervent belief that property law ought to be able to vindicate the value of community. The force of his belief is evident in the following passage from his reasons:

> But what has happened over the years between U.S. Steel, Youngstown and the inhabitants? Hasn't something come out of that relationship, something that out of which—not reaching for a case on property law or a series of cases but looking at the law as a whole, the Constitution, the whole body of law, not only contract law, but tort, corporations, agency, negotiable instruments—taking a look at the whole body of American law and then sitting back and reflecting on what it seeks to do, and that is to adjust human relationships in keeping with the whole spirit and foundation of the American system of law, to preserve property rights. . . . *[I]t seems to me that a property right has arisen from this lengthy, long-established relationship between United States Steel, the steel industry as an institution, the community of Youngstown, the people of the Mahoning Valley in having given and devoted their lives to this industry.*[21]

Following a full hearing, however, the district judge found himself unable to accord the union and community a property right in the mills. While he stated his continued belief that U.S. Steel ought not to be permitted to devastate the Youngstown community by closing the plants, he held that there was no authority on which he could found a property right in the community to prevent this from happening.[22] With much regret, therefore, the court found for U.S. Steel.

The Court of Appeals for the Sixth Circuit, in dealing with the appeal, also expressed deep sympathy for the plight of the Youngstown community.[23] The appeals court found itself in the same position, however, as had the district court: it could find no authority to support the grant of a property right to the community.[24] The court therefore held that it could offer the Youngstown community no assistance. In its opinion, only the legislature could resolve all the policy issues surrounding the question of plant closings.[25]

The *U.S. Steel* case is one in which strong noneconomic values supported the recognition of a community property right in the mills while economic values militated against such a recognition. Without the steel mills, Youngstown was in desperate shape. Not only were some 13,000 jobs lost as a result of the closings,[26] but the focus of the community was lost. With a property right to the mills, the community would have been able to force U.S. Steel to sell them the mills or, at least, to help establish some other industry to take the place of the one founded on steel. Without such a property right, the community was unable to prevent the tragedy that befell it.

The goal of enhancing trade in goods, in this case steel mills, is best ensured, on the other hand, by withholding a property right from the community. Trade in mills requires clear title. If workers or members of the community can simply pick up a property interest in a plant by working at the plant or living nearby, then title to the plant will be uncertain. This will hurt trade in two ways. First, managers of a mill will never know to whom they are responsible. As individuals in the community amass proprietary interests in the mill, ownership in the mill will become increasingly diluted. It will become unclear to management from whom, among the mass of owners, they are to take instructions. Second, prospective purchasers will be wary of buying the plant for fear that the ostensible owners cannot actually convey full title.[27]

Trade is enhanced by encouraging individuals to create goods. The more goods that are created, the more there is to trade. Thus, trade is enhanced when individuals build mills. Individuals will not build mills, however, unless they know they will reap the financial rewards from doing so. Property rights provide such individuals with the security that they, to the exclusion of all others, will be able to profit from the mills that they construct. If, however, the community can gain competing property rights to mills, individuals will lose this security. They will thus be less willing to invest in the construction of steel mills. Individuals are also less likely to invest in a mill where they do not control how their investment will be used. Individuals who risk their capital want to ensure that this capital is used wisely. They therefore wish to control the use to which their money is put. If others gain property rights to one's mill, however, one not only must share the mill itself but one must also share control over its capital. This added risk discourages investment.

The *U.S. Steel* case thus provides a showdown between community and economic values. While the judges were emotionally pulled toward vindicating community values above market value, once engaged in property-law discourse, they opted to uphold economic over community values. The judges refused to grant a property right that would have encouraged what all the judges acknowledged to be socially useful conduct, the preservation of the Youngstown community, and agreed to uphold a property right—that of U.S. Steel to the mills—that all understood would lead to socially harmful conduct, the devastation of Youngstown.

One can now see that when the received learning speaks of property as a label connoting the legal conclusion that something is valuable,[28] it is talking of market value. If other, noneconomic, values were included in the calculation of what is considered valuable, then the result in *U.S. Steel* would have been different.[29] Despite believing that the community interest in the mills was valuable in some sense, the judges deciding *U.S. Steel* did not believe that this interest was valuable in the sense employed in property discourse. The community interest was not economically valuable.

The community and the courts could, of course, have made some quasieconomic argument in favor of finding a community property right in the mills. One could have argued, for example, that U.S. Steel failed to consider the external costs of the shutdown of the mills. The decision was thus inefficient. If U.S. Steel were made to pay for this external cost, the argument could have gone, then U.S. Steel would only have shut down its mills if it were economically efficient to do so in those circumstances. Economic efficiency results in the best use of resources and maximizes trade. Granting a property right to the community in the mills would force U.S. Steel to buy out the community interest in the mills at a price that would compensate the community for the external costs. This would lead to an efficient result and would thus maximize trade. The grant of property rights in these circumstances would thus achieve the goal of property discourse: the promotion of economic values.

Such an argument, while at first appealing, so contradicts the premise of a market economy that one could not seriously put it forward as the basis for the award of property rights to the Youngstown community in the two steel mills. From an economic standpoint, the external costs of U.S. Steel's decision to close the plants—the loss of employment to the displaced workers, the loss of income to the city, the loss of trade to local businesses, and the ensuing loss of nonmill jobs—are nothing more than the losses incurred by individuals who took a risk and lost. Those who moved to Youngstown, those who took jobs at the mills, and those who established businesses in the city did so with the hope of making a living but at the risk that Youngstown would not survive. Each of these individuals made independent decisions as to the benefits they hoped to reap and the risks they were willing to take. They must, therefore, accept the consequences of their decisions, whether adverse or favorable. U.S. Steel, not having made these decisions, should not, on economic grounds at least, be held liable for these consequences.

The external costs of U.S. Steel's decision to shut down the plants are not, according to this analysis, external costs at all; they are simply the direct costs incurred by each member of the community in deciding to live or work in Youngstown. The national economy only works efficiently when all players benefit or lose according to the decisions they have made as to opportunity and risk. Placing additional burdens on individuals leads to inefficient results; such individuals will invest less than is optimal. When one attempts to hold U.S. Steel responsible for the costs incurred by others—specifically, by members of the Youngstown community—one risks inefficiency; U.S. Steel may decide to keep its inefficient and obsolete plants open instead of building efficient new ones. While this may temporarily please the inhabitants of Youngstown, the economy of the nation will suffer in the long term.

Without a plausible economic argument on which to rely, the Youngstown community could not, as had Monty Python, erect market values as a facade for its noneconomic interests. So, like the would-be immigrant to Germany who cannot pretend to be a refugee,

Youngstown was left out in the cold. While their interest in the well-being of their community was as strong or stronger than was the interest of Monty Python in its work, the citizens of Youngstown were left with no apparent means by which to vindicate that interest.

Confronted by the fact that it had only a noneconomic argument when property law appeared to require an economic one, the Youngstown community attempted to convince the court of appeals that the court was competent to consider noneconomic values in deciding whether to award the community a property right in the mills. The community relied on one sentence from the United States Supreme Court decision in *Munn v. Illinois*:[30] "So, too, in matters which do affect the public interest, and as to which legislative control may be exercised, if there are no statutory regulations upon the subject, the courts must determine what is reasonable."[31] In that case, the Illinois legislature set minimum grain storage charges in Chicago and other large cities in the state. The *Munn* court made the quoted statement in the course of affirming the state's authority to impose such minimum charges. The Youngstown community argued that, given the lack of legislative guidance in the area of community ownership of manufacturing plants, the court had to consider all values, not simply market values, inhering in the mills before making its determination.

The *U.S. Steel* court rejected Youngstown's argument that courts were competent to address noneconomic as well as economic arguments in deciding property-law cases. The court held that the *Munn* statement provided an insufficient basis for the court to order U.S. Steel to continue the operation of the two mills despite their unprofitability. The court noted that the United States had faced a long history of plant shutdowns. Determining how to respond to such shutdowns, the court held, implicated a great number of policy questions that courts are institutionally incompetent to consider. For this reason, it refused to consider Youngstown's claim that it needed a property right in the mills in order to uphold the value of community.[32]

Reductionalism to Economic Value

Given the myriad possible modes of valuing goods, there is no *a priori* reason why property discourse should limit itself to valuing goods in terms of market value. However, within property discourse it is assumed that this mode of evaluation necessarily encompasses all others. That is, courts seek to protect what they see as the common good through the allocation of property rights. They do so with the background belief that the market generally provides for this common good. That is, by placing goods into the market, courts assume that the market will put those goods to their highest use. The market achieves this result, according to the belief, because individuals place a money value on the way in which they value a particular good. The individual who values the good the most will be willing to pay the most for it. This individual will come to own the good, as she or he will outbid all other contenders. Given that this individual most values the good, she or he will put it to its highest use.

Notice also that the courts' understanding of the interaction of property rights and economic efficiency is a rather naive one. In none of the cases examined within the previous few chapters did a court take any serious step to determine whether, in fact, an efficient market in the contested good existed. That is, even accepting the hypothesis that the market does, in general, find a good's highest use, the courts failed to examine whether externalities or significant transaction costs existed that may have indicated market failure. This differentiates what the courts do in property cases from what economists suggest ought to be done. The latter would allocate property rights so as to minimize transaction costs. In other words, a more sophisticated economic analysis would attempt to allocate initial property rights in a good to that individual who values it the most.[33] This reduces the likelihood that transaction costs would prevent the efficient distribution of goods. Similarly, a more sophisticated economic analysis of property rights would seek to allocate such rights in such a manner designed to minimize enforcement costs and externalities.[34]

In addition to being naive, the courts' use of economic analysis has often been highly manipulative. As *Gilliam* illustrates, courts, when sympathetic to the actual values at stake, are content to support a property claim as long as they are presented with a plausible economic argument. What differentiated *Gilliam* from *U.S. Steel* was that in the latter no such argument was forthcoming. Presumably, given the district judge's comments at the pretrial hearing and the court of appeals's stated sympathy for the community, the *U.S. Steel* courts would have bent economic analysis somewhat to accommodate the community if such an argument had been presented. But a willingness to bend tradition is not the same as a willingness to break with it. Property discourse must be paid its dues.

The common good becomes, in property-law discourse, the encouragement of economic modes of valuation and faith in the market. Under this understanding of property, the quest to determine which activities ought to be promoted by property law is reduced to the calculation of market value and the promotion of trade. This has important implications for those who desire property rights in order to vindicate noneconomic values. Some of these implications will be discussed in chapters 8 and 9. We have seen, however, that one practical implication of this, as illustrated by *Gilliam* and *U.S. Steel*, is that one must present one's property claim on the basis of market value and the promotion of trade. When making one's argument, reliance on the value with which one is, in reality, concerned, is a poor strategy.

This chapter ends our foray into property discourse and property case law. This foray has illustrated that property discourse, as presently conceived, is premised on market price being the universal language of value and the market being the neutral arbiter of value. It is arguable, as discussed in chapter 9, that legal practitioners, in formulating property discourse, have misconceived the nature of property and the way property rights ought to be allocated. Despite the merits of any such argument, it is property discourse as practiced, and not as it ought to be, that will govern the way courts and legal practitioners argue about the appropriate allocation in goods. We must therefore ask ourselves whether property discourse as practiced is an appropriate vehicle through which to allocate rights of control over human biological materials.

To allocate property rights on the basis of economic modes of valuation is not to allocate those rights on the basis of noneconomic modes of valuation, although in any particular case both modes of valuation may result in the same allocation. To allocate a good to a person who will use or appreciate it in accordance with economic modes of valuation may be, as some of the cases examined in the last few chapters illustrate, inconsistent with its use or appreciation in noneconomic ways. When claims collide, property discourse favors granting rights to those who will put a good to economic use rather than to some noneconomic purpose.

Here, at its heart, is the result of the application of property discourse to goods: by allocating a good to those who value it in terms of economic modes of valuation, the good will be put to different purposes than it would have been put had we allocated it on the basis of noneconomic modes of valuation. The concern explored throughout this book over which modes of valuation we encourage through our application of property discourse is more than of merely academic concern; this concern goes to the ways in which we use goods in society. Unless we are ambivalent about human biological materials and the purposes to which they are put, we must ensure that we find some means of allocating rights of control over these materials so as to do justice to all of the ways that we value them.

While not all of us participate in the elucidation of property discourse, all of us are affected by it. Once rights of control are allocated through the application of property discourse by those sanctioned to apply it, the rest of the community must live with the outcome of that allocation. If the market does not function to ensure that the good to which the rights are granted ends up in the hands of that person who values it the most or if there is no method by which we can determine who values the good the most, then the good will not serve the highest purposes to which it can be put. To the extent that this occurs, we are all poorer, as that which has particular value, noneconomically speaking, will be put to purposes that very well may ignore that value. This flattening of the value landscape makes life that much less interesting and rich.

In the next three chapters, I return to an examination of the ways that we value human biological materials and whether there exists some way that we can both participate in property discourse and ensure that human biological materials are appropriately valued. Chapter 7 will highlight what is at stake in our decisions concerning the appropriate allocation of rights of control over human biological materials by illustrating some of the many ways that we, in this society, value these materials, the bodies from which they derive, and human health. Once I have presented how we, in fact, value these goods, I turn in chapter 8 to examine the question of whether the various ways that we value these goods can be either translated into some other value, such as market value, or ranked on some scale of value. Concluding that values are not translatable one into another and that there exists no common scale of value on which to rank them, I ask in chapter 9 whether, despite the faults of property discourse, it can be supplemented by other discourses that will directly take into account noneconomic modes of valuing human biological materials.

The conclusion I reach in these chapters is that property discourse seriously distorts how those employing it view those goods we call property. This is especially true for those goods, such as human biological materials, in which significant nonmarket values inhere. The consequence of such distortion is that, when there is a dispute over the use of the good, courts are unable to adequately weigh and consider the various values inhering in it. Their determination of rights thus threatens to ignore or discourage noneconomic modes of valuation.

7

Diverse Values in the Body and in Health

> On Vancouver Island, Ruth Benedict tells us, the Indians
> staged tournaments to measure the greatness of their princes.
> The rivals competed by destroying their belongings. They
> threw their canoes, fish oil, and salmon eggs on the fire, and
> from a high promontory, hurled their cloaks and pots into the
> sea.
> Whoever got rid of everything, won.[1]

The way each of us values the goods around us is complex, occasionally counterintuitive, and often conflicting. As the story recited by Ruth Benedict illustrates, one may value goods both instrumentally—as a means of transportation, as a source of nutrients, or as a way to stay warm—and intrinsically—as a symbol of community, competition, or power. Our appreciation of a good may change, for example, from valuing it as a means to prepare dinner to valuing it as a way to demonstrate political power.

Charles Taylor invokes the metaphor of a landscape when describing how we make decisions in relation to the goods that surround us.[2] According to Taylor, we make determinations within a moral landscape, or "framework," the features of which are the values that we hold.[3] How we place ourselves within that landscape and how we orient ourselves with respect to those values defines, in large part, who we are. In this landscape, some features appear more prominent or closer to us than do others; these are the values that are most important or most implicated in the decision before us. When we interact with a good—when we make a decision about that good—we do so within the framework of this landscape. For example, in Ruth Benedict's story, while the values of warmth and political power both featured within each prince's framework, the value of political power was the more prominent at the time each prince decided to throw his cloak over the cliff.

This chapter begins the task—one that I will not attempt to complete—of setting out some of the more prominent features in the moral landscape relating to the human body and human health. I set out the symbolic and metaphorical meaning of the body and of health in the realms of politics, individual development, religion, and superstition. This will set the groundwork for the discussion to follow in chapters 8 and 9 about whether property discourse is the appropriate vehicle to traverse this terrain.

The concept of individual frameworks implies that frameworks vary not only from person to person within a given culture—a culture based on shared beliefs and values—but even more so between cultures.[4] Therefore, I do not claim that those features of the moral landscape relating to the human body and human health that I lay out apply to all people or all cultures equally.[5] I, therefore, restrict my analysis to contemporary American society.

Once I have described the more prominent of those features within our moral landscape relating to the body and health, I set out three examples that I will use in chapter 8 to explore whether property discourse aids us in our travels through this landscape, at least with respect to making decisions about the human body and human health.

This chapter marks our return to the discussion of human biological materials. The function of this chapter is to lay out the context in which to evaluate the appropriateness of property discourse as it relates to the body and health, rather than to argue whether this discourse is appropriate. The conclusion I reach at the end of this chapter is that the way we view and understand the body and health is rich, complicated, and implicates many values, most of which are of a noneconomic variety.

The Body and Its Values

The human body reflects the society in which it exists. Social customs and institutions shape, or mark, the body directly (for example, through hairstyle, the piercing of ears, the removal of facial hair, and makeup) and indirectly (for example, through posture, facial expression, intonation, and scent). The body, according to Michel

Foucault,[6] is not so much refined as molded by social institutions such as the family, the school, the church, the workplace, and the community. According to this view, one cannot fully describe the human body apart from the society in which it exists.[7] In trying to understand the signification of the human body—what we understand the body and its components to mean—one must analyze the body within the context of a given society. As institutions and ideologies change, one should expect changes in the symbolic meaning of the body. The body as symbol comes to reflect these ideologies and institutions. Thus the female body, for example, in a sexist culture comes to symbolize passivity, weakness, and uncleanliness.[8] The religious injunction to forgive becomes the symbol of turning the other cheek.

The Body and Politics

In Western societies, the human body has taken on various meanings within the political realm. The body of the Middle Ages was an organic whole reflecting both the cosmological[9] and the political[10] orders. This body was harmonious, proportional, monumental, and male.[11] Within the Christian understanding of this time, the community of the faithful was considered to be the body of which Christ was the head.[12] This metaphorical use of the body symbolized the hierarchy within society: the head representing Christ, the eyes symbolizing the Church, the chest and arms denoting lay power, and the lower limbs and extremities corresponding to the masses.[13]

In the modern era, this organic view of the body gave way to a mechanical understanding of the body. No longer was the body a sacred incarnation of cosmological truth; rather, it was a worldly machine that could be made transparent through technology.[14] The modern body was an isolated unit no longer connected to the cosmos. Within the body, each organ performed its function in isolation. The then-current understanding of the body was therefore a reductionalist one. With increasing knowledge, this reduction went further, from organ, to cell, to gene.

This change of perspective led to the view that society was not a single body, but was composed of separate bodies whose relationship to one another was contingent.[15] The life of the individual, and no longer the life of the body politic, was paramount. The laborer, who had previously been metaphorically understood as the legs of the body politic, became an individual body like every other individual body in society, whether that of a member of the nobility, of the bourgeoisie, or of the laboring class.[16] The fact that each of us is embodied in similar bodies led to the replacement of a hierarchy of people with an equality of bodies. Each body within society was the equal of every other.

The signification of the human body is once again under transformation. As we in contemporary society have accumulated knowledge about the body and its workings, we have discovered that the reductive approach inherent in the mechanistic model is insufficient. Organs, cells, and genes do not, in fact, act in isolation; rather, their operation depends on how other organs, cells, and genes are functioning.[17] Pollution affects our bodies through the action of the environment—leading, for example, to allergies, asthma, and cancer—through the breakdown of the ozone layer—leading to skin cancer and cataracts—and through social interaction—leading to stress, heart disease, and sexually transmitted disease. We increasingly view the body as "a self-regulatory system whose functioning is dependent on, and inseparable from, the larger world, and which consequently can exist only in continuous, psychologically mediated interaction with a complex field of social, cultural, historical, and environmental conditions."[18]

The Body, Culture, and Self-Definition

Culture, like the political sphere of human life, imprints itself upon the body. Culture both marks the body and uses the body to express cultural beliefs. Culture directly marks the body through posture, walking gait, accent, and facial expressions. For example, British children are said to learn to hold their eyebrows in a raised position within their first few months of life.[19] Such cultural marks on the body forever associate the individual with the culture of his or her birth or development. In a similar manner, one's status within society is marked upon the body. Not only Eliza Doolittle's accent, but her posture and manner of walking had to be altered so that she could pass as an aristocrat. Similarly, caste marks, clothing, and hairstyles all display the wearer's place and status within society.

Just as the body is a symbol of cultural boundary, it is also a symbol of the boundary between individuals. Our bodies help to delineate the "me" from the surrounding universe. The infant's discovery of itself occurs, according to Jacques Lacan, at the moment the infant recognizes its body in a mirror.[20] When an infant reaches the "mirror stage," he or she for the first time understands that the image in the mirror is him or herself. At this instant, the infant becomes a subjective being. That is, by recognizing its body as its self, the infant becomes a subject, a human individual. And by associating its own body with "me," the infant comes to recognize the existence of others; for the only way to recognize itself as a distinct entity is for the infant to differentiate its body, and hence itself, from others.[21]

What is within the boundary of the self is very different from what is outside of this boundary. For example, there is an immense difference between saliva in our mouths and saliva we have spit out. While we would unhesitatingly swallow the former, we are generally loathe to swallow the latter.[22] Moreover, the boundary between what is "us" and what is not is far from clear and does not necessarily depend on the contours of our material body. Consider, for example, seating arrangements on a subway car, bus, or train. People seem to naturally space themselves out over the seats, each respecting the "space" around the others. We generally consider it rude to sit close to another person when there is open seating available. On the other hand, when a subway car is crowded, one feels little discomfort when someone not only sits near to one but actually touches one's body. Consider also the situation of someone bumping into your briefcase or umbrella. It would not seem at all unnatural for that person to say, "I'm sorry for bumping into you." Thus, the boundary between "us" and what is not us is not only unclear, but varies according to place and conditions.

Further, the boundary between what is us and what is outside need not correspond with the outside of the physical body. In Melanesia, for example, food is thought to contain the essence of the person who grew it. Thus, if someone were to surreptitiously bespell or burn someone else's food, the body of the person who grew the food is thought to suffer.[23] When an arm or leg is amputated, the amputee often still considers the lost limb as part of himself or herself. Thus, a pyrophobic patient may become truly fearful when the amputated limb is cremated.[24] The boundary between us and the surrounding world can even occur within the body proper. For example, Dr. Oliver Sacks describes a patient who failed to recognize his own leg as part of himself.[25]

The body is implicated far beyond this first differentiation of the "me" from the "they." It helps to shape each individual's understanding of her or himself and her or his place within society. For example, Hegel suggests that the will is alive in the body and this state of being is the precondition for every mode of existence,[26] from the individual, to the family, to society, to the state, and ultimately to world history. The human body is thus intrinsically valuable as the paradigmatic expression of the will in the external sphere. It is also instrumentally valuable as the precondition to every mode of existence. Each individual values her or his body as the embodiment of freedom and as the vehicle through which she or he senses the external world.[27] To others, the body of a person is what they recognize as that person.

Alternatively, drawing on the learning of Michel Foucault, we could say that we in society value human bodies as the site of the development of the "self." The body is the raw material for social forces that act upon it to form our conceptions both of the body and of the soul.[28] In this view, the body is socially created, shaped by power and knowledge relations. In contradistinction to the Hegelian framework, the body is not valued as the embodiment of the soul's freedom, but is seen as the prisoner of the soul.

The Body and Ritual

The body figures prominently in solemnization rituals. Marriage, for example, was traditionally consummated by sexual intercourse. In this way, the married couple was thought to become one flesh.[29] The body also symbolically formalizes other ceremonies. In the Old Testament, for example, important vows were formalized by placing the hand under the thigh.[30] Contemporary Western society continues to rely on body symbolism to formalize its rituals. Handshakes seal a deal[31] and one can ensure that one is being told the truth if the speaker looks one in the eye.

Less formal initiation rituals greet newborns in Western and other societies. Parents, grandparents, aunts, uncles, and friends each examine the newborn to determine whether the infant's nose more closely resembles that of the father or the mother, whether the baby has the grandfather's or grandmother's eyes, or whether the child's smile takes after one side of the family or the other. In this way, the physical characteristics of the child link him or her to past generations and situate the infant within a larger social group.

Funerals represent another important ceremony that centers on the body. By honoring the deceased's body, we pay homage to the deceased. Thus, we construct tombs to house the corpses of our great leaders, from kings and queens to Napoleon and Lenin. We also preserve parts of the deceased's body as relics. One of Galileo's fingers is, for example, on display in a museum in Florence. Similarly, hair from the deceased was collected in the nineteenth century as a memorial.

Relics from the bodies of saints have been particularly venerated. Umbrian peasants, around 1000, are recorded to have wished to kill Saint Romuald in order to make sure his bones would not be lost.[32] At the death of Saint Thomas Aquinas, the Fossanuova monks decapitated, boiled, and preserved the saint's body. While Saint Elizabeth of Hungary was lying in state in 1231, worshippers cut off parts of her body to preserve them as relics. Similarly, at the funeral of the Ayatollah Khomeni, some of the faithful tore at his body in order to possess a relic.[33]

This tradition of collecting relics from the dead continues in Western culture, albeit in a different form. Instead of preserving a finger or some hair from the deceased, we now collect photographs. Photographs, being a representation of the body of the deceased, more than letters or drawings, serve the same purpose as did relics in the past: they help us remember and honor our ancestors. Whether we look at them often or infrequently, photographs are among our most precious treasures. This is perhaps why, for example, following the death of a loved one, it is not uncommon for a family to lovingly peruse the deceased's collection of photographs and to distribute them equitably among family members.

Rituals of sharing also involve the body. In his expansion upon an argument credited to Richard Titmuss,[34] Thomas Murray argues that gifts of the body—for example, blood and kidneys—to strangers affirm the "quintessentially human"[35] gift of solidarity. "Blood represents individual life and vitality, and at the same time it signifies the oldest, most primitive tie that affirms solidarity and binds people to one another." Within this understanding, the body, or, more precisely, the donation of a part of the body, is valuable because it promotes solidarity in society.

The Sacred Body and the Profane Body

Perhaps the area in which the human body has its richest symbolism is in connection with that which is sacred and that which is profane. The human body is an earthly reflection of the divine; according to Western religions, our bodies are made in the image of God.[36] At the same time, the body symbolizes the profane. For example, giving into one's "fleshly" desires or one's appetites is often considered a sin.

Blood is accorded a sacred place among the body's components. Blood is associated with life itself; when God bade Noah to be fruitful and multiply and to eat every living thing, God forbade the consumption of blood. "Only you shall not eat flesh with its life, that is, its blood. For your lifeblood I will surely require a reckoning; of every beast I will require it and of man."[37]

Blood has been granted the ability to speak for the deceased after death. Thus, Abel's blood spoke to God with news of Abel's murder.[38] In Medieval Northern Albania, a bottle of a victim's blood was watched by kin to see if it "boiled," or fermented. If the blood did boil, vengeance was immediately taken; otherwise, compensation for the death was accepted.[39] Similarly, among some Melanesian peoples, the corpse or the corpse's blood was thought to indicate whether the deceased had died naturally or through sorcery.[40]

Parallel to the body's representation of the sacred, the body symbolizes the profane. In Christian belief, the body signifies both sin and dirt. Thus, to remove the taint of original sin, the body must be ritually bathed in baptism. The metaphorical link between sin and dirt is continued through the foot-washing ceremony. Once cleansed (baptized) of dirt (sin), the body (soul) need only be cleansed where it touches the earth (vice). Thus, Jesus taught that "[h]e who has bathed does not need to wash except for his feet, but he is clean all over."[41]

Through self-flagellation and fasting, religious ascetics attempt both to transcend the body (sin) and to mark their body as holy.[42] The pain of self-flagellation, because of its excruciating intensity, blocks out worldly demands, leaving the penitent alone with God.[43] The fast purifies the "abominable" stomach so that it can receive the holy host of the Eucharist.[44] Both practices physically mark the body of the ascetic, through scars and an anorexic body that speak of the ascetic's holiness.[45]

The female body, in particular, has been associated with the profane. In Western culture, women have been variously labeled as sexually insatiable,[46] as imperfect,[47] and as grotesque.[48] The belief in the profanity of the female body has worked itself into beliefs concerning conception. According to one such belief, while the female body was given credit for the formation of the material parts of the fetus, the male body was thought to contribute the more important form or essence of the child. According to Aristotle, for example, the father's semen, instead of being made of lowly earth, was thought to be made from water and air. Aristotle believed that semen contributed only form to the growing body; the material substance of the child was left to the mother.[49] This same dichotomy between idea and matter is well illustrated in the story of Jesus's conception. Jesus is conceived through the ethereal contribution of the Holy Spirit and the material contribution of Mary.[50] The profanity of the female body is somewhat alleviated in this case because Mary was a virgin, the least profane of female bodies.

Sin itself has been thought to mark the body. Red hair has been associated with the presence of the devil, while green eyes are said to be a sign of jealousy. To punish Eve for eating the apple from the tree of knowledge, God inflicted the pain of childbirth upon women's bodies.[51] Similarly, Cain's body was marked by God as a sign both of Cain's guilt and that none should kill Cain.[52] The belief that sin marks the body is tragically demonstrated today by those who preach that AIDS is a punishment from God for immoral sexual conduct.[53]

The profane nature of the human body is not always condemned, however. In fact, the sexuality of the body, principally the female body, is heightened through clothing, makeup, and hairstyles. High-heeled shoes, for example, emphasize hip movement and cause both buttocks and chest to protrude.[54] Similarly, cosmetics accentuate the eyes, increasing sexual attractiveness. To a lesser extent, men's clothing also enhances sexual appeal; shoulder pads enhance the appearance of upper body strength while neckties serve as a phallic symbol.

The symbolism of the human body, which this chapter has only cursorily explored, is rich and varied within Western culture. The body signifies the relation between individual and world, individual and state, and the sacred and the profane. While some have argued that there is no *a priori* reason for according the body a prominent position in our understanding of ourselves and our world,[55] it appears to be a contingent truth that every human culture invests the body with deep symbolic meaning. Our bodies symbolically link us to our ancestors, our community, and our children. Our understanding of our own identity is profoundly influenced by our bodies and the meanings we attach to them.

Human Health

The way we value human health overlaps, for obvious reasons, with the way we value the human body. Because health describes a state of the body (although a highly ambiguous and, as I will discuss, culturally contingent one), many of the values identified in the foregoing discussion of the body apply to human health. Nonetheless, health and the body are distinct goods. Health relates not only to the physical body, but to the mind; it denotes not so much the ideal of a perfect body but a state of relative lack of illness. Unlike the body, health cannot be seen, although it may be perceived. It is described not by what it is, but what it is not—the absence of illness, suffering, and pain.

Health and Politics

Health is both a metaphor for politics and a metaphor used in politics to justify or support the doing of certain actions. We often discuss politics in terms of health. We say that one of the goals of politics is to "heal" rifts between communities. Racial intolerance, spousal assault, and other social "ills" are "open sores" in our society. Poverty and homelessness are said to be at "epidemic" levels.

We not only use the analogy between health and politics to give color to our description of politics, but we apply our understanding of health in order to understand politics. Politicians ask us "to take our medicine" in order to bring the economy back to "health." Capital punishment was understood, in the eighteenth century, as the political equivalent of amputation. At that time, capital punishment was seen as a "cure" for illness in the body politic.[56] Those who stole or murdered endangered the life of the body politic to the same extent as a gangrenous limb threatened the life of the human body. The remedy, in both cases, was amputation. By cutting off the ailing limb, health was restored both to the body politic and to the human body. Judges pronouncing sentences of death were, therefore, in the same position as physicians amputating legs; both were healing the sickness of the body.

The analogy between health and politics is also apparent in literature. Albert Camus in his book, *The Plague*,[57] uses a fictional plague devastating a French city as a metaphor for the Nazi occupation of France during World War II.[58] By viewing the Nazi occupation as a plague, Camus explores the political and bureaucratic reasons behind France's sudden fall to Germany, the lack of hope that Germany could be defeated, and the evolution, in the inhuman face of Nazism, of the Resistance into a militaristic and cutthroat force. The analogy between plague and Nazism works, in large part, because of the analogy between political community and the body; just as the human body may sometimes become ill and require unpleasant and painful medical attention, so too the body politic may occasionally become ill and require harsh and painful treatment in the hands of community leaders.

The Nazis themselves used the analogy between health and politics to further their program of genocide. The Nazis portrayed Jews, Slavs, and Gypsies as "racial parasites" who represented a health threat to Germany in that their genes would weaken the Aryan gene pool.[59] The medical analogy carried through to the death camps: the process of selection for those who would be sent to the gas chambers resembled medical triage; inmates undressed in "medical blocks" and were used for medical "experimentation."[60]

Another connection between health and politics is the notion that good citizenship requires that we keep ourselves in good health. This connection is currently illustrated in debates surrounding smoking, the wearing of seat belts in automobiles, and the wearing of bicycle helmets. Plato understood health to be a sound pattern of living.[61] Those who became ill, other than by reason of epidemic, were thought to have been morally irresponsible.

Health practitioners, while occupying a position of moral neutrality—they do not usually tell us what is morally right or wrong—dispense morally loaded diagnoses by labeling certain pains and certain conditions as illness while refusing to recognize others as such.[62]

This is a double-edged sword. If one's behavior is labeled "illness"—whether it be homosexuality or stress from an unsatisfying occupation—then many members of society, if not most, will view the behavior as a personal inconvenience or tragedy and not as a political statement. If one's behavior is not labeled "illness"—for example, if a physician says that a loved one did not kill him or herself because of a mental disability and thus committed "suicide" rather than died of an illness—one may be subjected to social sanction.[63]

Physicians not only exercise social control through the determination of which sets of conditions or symptoms amount to illness; they also exercise this control by discovering the cause, or etiology, of disease. The cause of disease is located within the patient's body rather than depending on environmental, occupational, social, or political circumstances.[64] Thus, instead of working to reduce occupational hazards, we counsel those who possess a susceptibility to particular illnesses to seek another job.[65] By looking at the patient's body to discover the etiology of disease, health care professionals place responsibility for disease on the patient. Individuals choose to take health risks, accept hazardous jobs, and live near polluted water; the social or environmental conditions leading to disease are not to blame.[66] By focusing on the individual rather than on the social, environmental, and political surroundings of the individual, medicine misses much. "Instead of examining the work conditions that create stress, attention is focused on how adequately the individual responds to stress. Instead of looking at the marital, family, or work pressures of a compulsive overeater or smoker, emphasis is placed upon the individual's will power to control personal behaviour."[67]

A third way that physicians exert social control is through the physician–patient relationship. A patient visiting a physician not only lacks the physician's expertise, but is anxious about the result of the encounter.[68] Physicians control the flow of information, both from the patient to the physician—through an interview process—and from the physician to the patient.[69] The nature of physical examinations may lead the patient to feel awkward, if not embarrassed.[70] Physicians concentrate on the efficient use of their time and try to avoid spending time with patients that they perceive to be contributing to their own illness by their lifestyle or their failure to accept treatment.[71] Physicians adopt a scientific approach to disease in which the causes of disease can be rationally explained; emotional or social aspects of a patient's illness are thus generally not of concern to the physician.[72] In adopting a scientific, rather than sociological, approach to disease, physicians tend to rely more on technology than on counseling or other nonintrusive measures and to express a concomitant concern for elongating life rather than improving quality of life.[73]

Health and Culture

What we understand to be health and our obligation to be healthy is dependent on our self-understanding. One's understanding of what it is to be healthy varies from culture to culture.[74] Thus, being in a particular state may be labeled "ill" by members of one ethnic group and not ill by members of another group or by the same group at another time. Our language reflects this change of labels; whereas once a person was considered "disabled" by a condition, whether physical or mental in origin, and thus unable to function in society as a full member, now that person is "challenged" by the condition.[75]

Most health care is provided by nonprofessionals in noninstitutional settings.[76] We self-administer dietary restrictions and medicine and curtail certain activity to stave off or treat illness. Other than self-care, family members and friends provide the bulk of health care services, such as providing food, changing dressings, administering medication, and monitoring symptoms. Which conditions at what point in their development we decide to pass on to health care professionals depends on such factors as whether we consider the condition abnormal or simply the result of too hectic a life; whether we believe the condition to be caused by nonphysical causes, such as emotions or spirits; and social expectations of how to deal with the condition.

A society's determination of how to deliver health services to its members also points to the role that the values of community and of sharing play within that society.[77] Where health services are granted to individuals as a right of citizenship, health is understood, at least in part, as the concern of the community rather than of the individual. On the other hand, where, as in the United States, no universal health coverage is available, the value of individualism is paramount.

Health, Spirituality, and Religion

Religious salvation also has strong metaphorical links to health and healing. "Salvation is basically and essentially healing, the re-establishment of a whole that was broken, disrupted, disintegrated."[78]

Jesus's ability to heal the blind, the lame, and lepers supported the claim that he was the Messiah.[79] Other myths of salvation similarly link salvation with bodily and cosmic health.[80]

The correspondence between grace and health on the one hand and between sin and illness on the other runs through Western history. In the Middle Ages, health represented the certainty of grace, while illness was thought to be a punishment or ordeal.[81] Later, poor teeth were thought to be a sign of sexual guilt.[82] In the last century, masturbation was both a sin and a cause of disease.[83] In literature, Dorian Gray's numerous sins marked his portrait with sores and scars.[84]

Many modern religious sects rely on their own understanding of health both to differentiate themselves from the rest of society and to exert control over their membership.[85] Alternatively, individuals have turned to an eclectic mixture of health and religious practices such as meditation, healing circles, and Western occult traditions in an effort to reconnect their minds, bodies, and spirits.[86] Rather than view one's health as the purely technical problem of identifying certain conditions and administering certain medicines, these individuals see a link between physical health, emotional health, spiritual health, and well-being that modern medicine seems to ignore. This view is supported by the feeling that physicians treat patients as objects with no say in their medical treatment and that physicians look too narrowly at the body for the sources of illness.[87]

Despite the obvious links between the human body and human health, each relates to its own distinct set of values within our frameworks of understanding. While the body is connected to the values of identity, community, sharing, and sin, human health is connected to the values of individual responsibility and political and moral control. Many of the issues involved in the question of the ownership of human biological materials implicate both sets of values. Thus whenever we make determinations about these materials, whether we are conscious of it or not, we decide which of these values to further and which to ignore.

Cell Lines: A Reprise of *Moore*

The subject matter of the property claim in *Moore* v. *Regents of the University of California*[88] was a cell line derived from the spleen of

Moore. Golde and the pharmaceutical companies considered the cell line valuable because it overproduced lymphokines in high enough quantities to harvest commercially. Unlike most cell lines, the cell line in dispute derived only from Moore. Therefore, despite their handling and induced ability to self-replicate, the cells in the cell line contained Moore's DNA.

The *Moore* court identified three values inhering in the cell line: Moore's dignity, his autonomy, and increased discovery of pharmaceuticals. Moore's dignity and autonomy were implicated in the decision to allocate control over the cell line because of the circumstances under which the cells were taken from his body: during a medical procedure without his knowledge of the possibility that the cells would be used for commercial gain. Moore did not have the opportunity either to refuse to share his cells with the community or to dedicate his cells to the good of the community. In this respect, the values of sharing and community were also at play.

The issue of autonomy arises in two respects. First, Golde treated Moore as an object on which to practice his technical expertise. He felt no need to disclose his commercial interest in Moore's cells to Moore, despite the commercial importance of the cells to him. In his view, Moore was merely a passive participant in the health care process.

Second, the values of autonomy and identity are together at play in the determination of how to treat the cells after their removal from Moore. Since the cells and Moore are linked by their shared DNA, Moore may have felt that the cells continued to be part of him following their removal. Thus, when Golde removed the cells from his body, Moore may have felt that part of himself had been taken away. Furthermore, Golde's continuing control over the fate of the cell line may, to Moore, have felt like continuing control over part of himself. This was likely exacerbated by the fact that Moore, at Golde's instructions, continued to provide Golde with blood, semen, and hair samples over an extended period following the splenectomy.

The *Moore* court's concern for the discovery of new pharmaceuticals implicates other values bound up with health care policy. The push for the discovery of new medicines implies a technological understanding of disease rather than one focused on community or spirituality. In addition, it is a reductionalist view of health care (in which the cause of illness is understood as located within the body of the patient), rather than a holistic view (in which disease is understood as the interactions among the patient, the environment, the workplace, and society).

It is difficult to balance all of these considerations. Many point to leaving control over the cell line in Moore's hands, while others point to giving that control to Golde. What can be gleaned from this short discussion is that the *Moore* court, in reaching its decision, did not weigh all of the values at stake nor explain how their decision would affect these values.

DNA Fragments

In June 1991 the National Institutes of Health filed patent applications on fragments of complementary DNA—DNA that has been reverse-engineered from expressed genes. This move was heavily criticized both in the United States and internationally. Many debated what effect the grant of these patents would have on the future development of biotechnologies. In February 1994 the National Institutes of Health withdrew these applications.

Human DNA occurs in long strands containing both expressed and unexpressed sequences.[89] Inside the cell, sequences of DNA are translated into RNA[90] strands that are then chopped to remove those sequences of RNA corresponding to the unexpressed DNA sequences. These messenger RNA strands are then translated into proteins. Complementary DNA (cDNA) is made by reversing the process by which DNA is translated into RNA. The resulting cDNA contains only the expressed portion of genes. An investigator at the National Institutes of Health found a method of quickly sequencing fragments of this cDNA. These sequenced fragments could then be used as tags to locate genes within longer segments of DNA.[91]

The skirmish over the attempt to patent cDNA fragments was fought on the basis of how best to encourage medical research. Those favoring the grant of patent rights argued that patent protection offered the necessary economic incentive to encourage researchers to develop drugs and other therapies; those arguing against the grant of patent rights held that the monopoly over the use of cDNA created by the patent would likely stifle basic research in medicine, thus lessening the chance that a new medical treatment would be discovered.[92]

The debate over the patentability of cDNA fragments ignored other values at stake. These include the values of community and of sharing. The DNA in each of our cells is, statistically, almost identical to the DNA in everyone else's cells. DNA thus represents a common heritage shared by the world community and demonstrates equality among individuals, at least at the molecular level. Like blood, which is common to all of us, the information contained in DNA is capable of being shared for our mutual benefit.

Control of cDNA also affects the values inhering in health. The use of cDNA in genetic research implicates both the sacred nature of human life and the fear of eugenics. The question of the extent to which it is permissible to alter human genetic material was not addressed in the debate over the patentability of cDNA.

Additionally, the enterprise of sequencing fragments of cDNA contributes to the reductionalism of health care. The attributes of an individual, whether good or bad, are looked for in that individual's genes rather than in the environment or workplace. We thus search for genes that lead to obesity, to violence, or to promiscuity.[93] The choice of health care policy implicit in the arguments on both sides of debate surrounding the patentability of cDNA fragments is that medicine ought to be reductionalist. This choice ignores, however, the desire demonstrated by those who embrace holistic medicine, traditional medicine, and the occult in an attempt to link mind, body, and spirit.

As was the case with the ownership of the cell line in *Moore*, the debate surrounding the patentability of cDNA fragments focused almost exclusively on only one of the many values that were at stake in the debate; both sides justified their position on the basis of the promotion of research with the aim of discovering and bringing to market new drugs and therapies. The issues of the cultural and social meanings of the body and health care and, more generally, the interaction between our frameworks of understanding and the body and health, were not discussed.

Organ Donation

Human organs can be transplanted from one individual to another in the right circumstances. Sometimes organs can only be taken from cadavers—such as hearts and lungs—and other times they can be donated by living individuals—for example, kidneys. Although the number of potentially suitable organs obtainable from cadavers is greater than the number of organs needed for transplantation, most of these organs are not donated.[94] Because of the shortage of available organs, individuals occasionally advertise to purchase an organ.

Some have argued that individuals ought to own their organs and be entitled to sell them on the market. The argument is that the economic incentive provided by the market will encourage people to sell their organs—either immediately or upon their death—and thus eliminate the shortage of available organs. This argument ignores other values inhering in these organs. These range from the sanctity of the human body, to respect for our ancestors, to sharing, and to community. Since we often identify ourselves with our bodies, the thought of cutting out pieces and giving them to others is uncomfortable to many. Further, to the extent that one believes the human body to be made in God's image, it may be sinful to cut open the body. On the other hand, if one is to part with something as close to our identity as an organ, many of us would prefer to do so out of a concern for community or altruism rather than for a money price. Donating an organ or blood is giving the gift of life. Once a market in the organ is introduced, however, it may feel as if the donation means no more than giving a gift of money.[95]

The issue of individual responsibility is also implicated in organ transplants. The patient may require the transplant because she or he may have smoked too much or drunk too much alcohol or may have been engaged in dangerous activities. On the other hand, the donation of an organ by one individual to another demonstrates communal concern over the health of each person.

These three examples illustrate that decisions involving the control or ownership of human biological materials implicate many disparate values within our frameworks of understanding in such various realms as the political, the individual, the communal, and the spiritual. Whether or not it consciously considers and weighs each of these values, when a court allocates property rights to human biological materials it effectively determines the topology and geography of our moral landscapes.

The previous chapters of this book have illustrated that, in allocating property rights to goods, courts aim at vindicating economic values; other values that may inhere in the good are presumed to be weighed and compared by the market. In applying this approach to human biological materials, courts are likely to award property rights to these materials on the basis that the market is in the best position to determine how these materials ought to be used. The courts will thus award property rights to the parties most likely to make an economic use of them. In doing so, values such as community, sharing, identity, and spirituality will be pushed aside. If these values are to be vindicated, then, they are to be vindicated through market forces. The next chapter examines whether the market is capable of fulfilling this function.

8

Translating Value

53. He who pierces an arm shall pay 6 shillings compensation.

    ¶1. If an arm is broken, 6 shillings shall be paid as compensation.

54. If a thumb is struck off, 20 shillings [shall be paid as compensation].

    ¶1. If a thumb nail is knocked off, 3 shillings shall be paid as compensation.

    ¶2. If a man strikes off a forefinger, he shall pay 9 shillings compensation.

    ¶3. If a man strikes off a middle finger, he shall pay 4 shillings compensation.

    ¶4. If a man strikes off a 'ring finger,' he shall pay 6 shillings compensation.

    ¶5. If a man strikes off a little finger, he shall pay 11 shillings compensation.[1]

Even if it be true that life is priceless, the same cannot be said of the human body. As the seventh-century law quoted here attests, societies have long attached a market price to body parts. This practice continues today when courts grant or insurers pay compensation for the loss of a hand, a foot, or an eye. Neither the courts nor the insured live under the illusion, however, that this money price actually captures the true value of a lost limb or organ. The price is not actually a price at all; it is merely a payment to enable the tort victim to get on with life and to sufficiently punish the wrongdoer so that he or she will not again be negligent.

    The law, in its various guises, constantly measures the value of the human body. Criminal law vindicates the value of autonomy by punishing those who injure or confine our bodies. Family law vindicates the value of physical safety and well-being by ensuring that those who care for children meet their physical needs. Labor law vindicates both autonomy and well-being through the establishment of maximum hours of work and health and safety standards. Insurance law vindicates the value of independence by providing individuals with a safety net should they be physically injured. Contract law vindicates moral values by holding immoral contracts, such as those for sexual services, to be unenforceable. The law of *habeas corpus* vindicates the value of dignity by ensuring that officials of the state do no harm to prisoners.

Courts, in dealing with various aspects of the human body, measure and compare the values inhering in it. To decide, for example, whether a "fair fight" is an assault under the criminal law, courts consider several values inhering in the human body. First, given that such a fight is likely to result in physical injury, the legality of the fight raises the value of safety. Second, because each of the participants in the fight consented to it—otherwise it would not have been a fair fight—the court must deal with the value of autonomy as it relates to the decision to enter into the fight. Third, since public brawls upset the peace of a community, the courts must consider the value of peace. Fourth, since many members of the public view any fight as immoral, the issue of morality is implicated. While the values of safety, peace, and morality are furthered by holding fair fights to be illegal, the value of autonomy is not. In determining whether and under what circumstances such a fight is a criminal assault, therefore, the court has to establish a satisfactory balance among these values.

The task of balancing the competing values inhering in a good can be a daunting one. Courts often attempt to avoid such balancing by holding themselves incompetent to consider any but a narrow set of values inhering in the good. Recall, for example, that the Court in *Diamond v. Chakrabarty*[2] held that it was incompetent to consider the values of health and safety that those opposed to the grant of patent rights in living organisms raised. Recall also that the court in *Local 1330, United Steel Workers of America v. United States Steel*[3] held that, despite the importance of the value of community, the courts could not vindicate this value. On the other hand, neither the *Chakrabarty* nor the *U.S. Steel* courts found any difficulty in considering the effects of their decision on economic values.

If one hopes to avoid the procrustean solution of ignoring

competing value claims, one must find an alternative to it. One alternative is to develop a method of comparing and ranking the various values implicated in a decision. If one could establish a single scale of value into which every other value could be translated, the courts would simply be able to place all implicated values on that scale and compare them. By measuring the importance of each implicated value on this scale and comparing it with the importance of every other value, the courts could easily determine how to maximize overall value. For example, consider the problem of determining whether one should buy apples by the bag or individually. Suppose each bag of apples costs two dollars per pound and each apple, sold in bulk, costs thirty-five cents. Assuming the apples are of the same quality and taste, how is one to choose which to buy? The most straightforward method to make one's decision is to find a common scale of value. For apples, that scale is price per given weight. Suppose that the bag of apples weighs two pounds and that, on average, four apples weigh one pound. Once one translates the cost of the bag and the bulk apples onto this scale, one easily discovers that one pound of bagged apples costs $1 while one pound of bulk apples costs $1.40. One therefore will choose to buy apples by the bag.

Therefore, one alternative to the unsatisfactory solution of ignoring certain values is to find a common scale of value on which one can compare and rank all of the values inhering in a particular good. When a court is faced with the decision of whether a fair fight is a criminal assault, it can simply place all values implicated in that decision on such a scale. It would then be a simple matter of adding up the values of safety, peace, and morality on one side and autonomy on the other and seeing which sum is greater. The court would simply make an order in favor of the side having the greater sum.

On a reconsideration of the cases examined throughout this book, one would soon see that the courts do, in fact, rely on a common scale of value in resolving property-law claims. This scale is market value. In the market, each individual attaches a market price to the way in which she or he values a particular good. Individuals attach higher prices to goods they value more strongly. For example, someone whose livelihood depends on a computer will be willing to pay more for a computer than someone who simply desires a computer for recreational use. In a free and open market, whoever currently holds a good will sell it to that individual who is willing to pay the most for it.[4] Since the latter most values the good, the market ensures that the good is used in such a fashion as to maximize overall value—as measured on the scale of market value.

This chapter explores whether the plethora of values inhering in the human body and human health explored in chapter 7 can be measured and compared on some common scale of value. Given that property discourse is founded on market value, previous chapters have illustrated that practitioners in making their arguments and courts in reaching their decisions acknowledge but a few of these values and directly consider the impact of their arguments on fewer still. This chapter examines whether, despite the lack of direct examination of noneconomic values, the market will appropriately weigh and compare these values indirectly. This discussion centers on whether the values are commensurable.

The discussion of commensurability ends with the conclusion that a common scale on which to rank values does not exist. Therefore, any reliance on market forces to further the values inhering in the human body and human health is misplaced. Courts cannot simply insert a good into the market with the expectation that the values inhering in that good will be considered and ranked. Simply because the market cannot rank values does not, however, mean that courts are helpless in making choices among values. Courts will have to undertake a direct examination of the values inhering in a good in order to select the most appropriate way in which to treat that good.

Commensurability

The cases discussed in previous chapters of this book support the conclusion that in their analysis of property-law claims centering on the human body, courts focus their inquiry on the question of whether granting property rights in the body or body parts furthers trade in the body and its parts; they do not examine whether the noneconomic values inhering in the human body and in human health are harmed or furthered through the allocation of property rights. The courts leave the furtherance of these values and the continued development of the social meaning of the body and health to the action of the market. They do so on the implicit assumption that the market appropriately measures and compares the various, often competing, values inhering in goods.

If the assumption that the market will appropriately weigh and compare values is correct, the courts are right in placing goods into the market. Instead of trying to accomplish the seemingly impossible task of considering all values and how their decisions will affect those values, the courts have only to turn over this task to the market. The market is, because of its vastness and its ability to reflect everyone's tastes—through the fact that every member of society participates in the market to some extent—in a much better position to undertake this task than are the courts. This logic is based, however, on the assumption that the market can and does measure and compare values.

The remainder of this chapter examines whether the assumption that the market can and does measure and compare values is correct. The assumption has two elements: first, that there exists some scale into which every value inhering in a good can be translated; and second, that this scale is money. For example, this assumption would hold that one's autonomy can be assigned a money value.

It would be sufficient for the purposes of the arguments advanced in this book to undermine the second of these assumptions, that money is a superscale of value, since this would demonstrate that any reliance on the market to rank values is ill-founded. But to simply make this argument leaves open the possibility that other superscales exist and that all one must do to meet the concerns expressed in this book would be to find a better superscale. This chapter concentrates, therefore, on the first part of the assumption, that no common superscale of value exists.

The issue of ranking values on a common scale comes to the fore most strongly where there are apparently conflicting values. Consider, for example, the disparate claims of scientific investigation and religious belief on the body. The body, from a scientific viewpoint, is a source of knowledge of physical development, aging, and disease. From a religious perspective, the body is understood as a sacred object, being created in the image of God. The scientist values the body instrumentally, as a means to acquire knowledge; the believer values the body intrinsically, for being an image of God. Within the framework of understanding of each of the scientist and the believer, the body is valued in an appropriate manner. It is only when the frameworks of scientist and believer make disparate claims upon the body that a conflict arises, one that is not obviously resolvable within either framework. Such a conflict could occur if, for example, the scientist wishes to perform an autopsy, which the believer holds to be a violation of the body's sacred nature, on a cadaver.

If it were either true that the understanding of the scientist could be translated into the language of the believer (or vice versa), or true that both the language of the scientist and that of the believer could be translated into a metalanguage, then the apparent conflict between scientist and believer could be resolved within this all-encompassing language. In other words, if the values of scientist and of believer were commensurable—that is, could be ranked on a single common scale of value—the conflict would turn out to be more apparent than real. While disputes would not be eliminated, since people would continue to have imperfect understanding based on incomplete information, they would, in principle, be resolvable.

Valuing Color

To help understand, by analogy, the claim that values are commensurable, consider the following interpretation of color perception.[5] Normal human color vision is based on red, green, and blue light. That is, cone cells in our eyes are activated by either red, green, or blue light. Imagine looking at an object that causes our red, green, and blue cones to fire in a certain proportion (B units of red, D units of green, and F units of blue in Figure 1). Our brains register these various units of red, green, and blue, and determine that the object is a certain color (point H in Figure 1). Call this last color simply "color."

With this example in mind, we may ask whether colors are commensurable. That is, can the colors of different objects be placed upon a common scale and ranked? It must first be noted that one cannot simply compare measurements of red, green, and blue on a common scale. If we could, then B units of red, D units of green, and F units of blue would equal D units of red, F units of green, and B units of blue, which they clearly do not. (This would be equivalent to saying that a certain hue of brown is equal to a certain hue of purple.) Such a statement is meaningless since no one with color vision could make sense of it.

One can attempt to commensurate color in various ways. First, one can take one of the three sense perceptions that go into the determination of color—that is, the firing of either red, green, or blue cones in the eyes—to be the one really authentic perception of color and then compare colors based on that perception. (This is similar to the hedonist suggestion that we take one good, pleasure, and rank

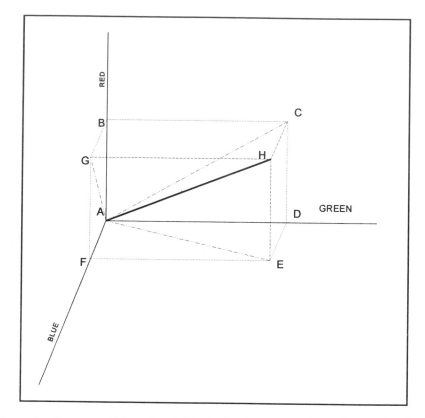

Figure 1. Every possible color visible to the human eye is a mixture of red, green, and blue light. This figure describes all possible colors three-dimensionally, with red corresponding to the vertical axis, green the horizontal axis, and blue the forward axis. Each color is represented by a point in this space with the origin, point A, being black. In order to place point H on a scale of "colorfulness," we must be able to assign some fixed value to color H, for example, the distance in color space between black (point A) and the point H. The length of line AH, while permitting us to rank different colors in an abstract sense, does not reflect the subjective feeling of the color corresponding to point H. It does not, therefore, permit us to rank the subjective feeling corresponding to each color.

all other goods in terms of it.) That is, one can reduce color determination to one common factor, say green, and simply determine whether a particular color is more or less green than another. If one wants to maximize color, one can simply choose the most "green" object (the one that has the most units of green in it). In Figure 1, for example, the color corresponding to point H has D units of green.

While reducing color to the firing of green cones has the advantage of commensurating colors, it does so at the loss of much that is interesting about color: the redness, blueness, and the combination red–blueness. Some of this richness can be restored if we measure all color in terms of, for example, red–greenness (point C in Figure 1). This, however, not only fails to capture all there is about color, specifically its blueness, but it does not even provide a meaningful standard against which to measure color. While we do know that B units of red and D units of green is greater than B units of red by itself, is it equal, greater, or less than D units of red and B units of green?

A more propitious tack would be to find a common scale outside of the firings of red, green, or blue cones in the eye. For example, one can simply calculate the length of line AH in Figure 1. This length can be measured against the length of any other color to determine whether one color is greater, equal, or less than the other. Since the length of AH depends on all cone firings, and not simply on one type, such as the firings of green cones, it captures the richness of color. Notice further that the scale on which the length AH—call this the color superscale—is measured has no counterpart in the world. That is, nowhere in the process of determining color does the length AH figure; the brain determines color from the raw data of red, green, and blue cone firings, without ever calculating the length AH. Thus, while the measurement of the line AH captures some of the complexity of color, it does not, in any meaningful way, correspond to the sensory perception of color. The ranking of one color ahead of another based on the measurement of AH is an artifice that, while providing one way to talk about color, does not in any way correspond to the way we feel or think about color.[6]

The Lack of a Metascale

Unfortunately, the enterprise of attempting to rank color on some metascale, such as the measurement of the line AH, is a hopeless one. The determination of the color of an object depends not merely on the number of red, green, and blue cone firings occurring in the eye, but on the surface properties of the object, general lighting conditions, and the color of nearby objects.[7] Painters have long known that altering the juxtaposition of pigments on a canvas changes one's determination of what colors one sees. Photographers constantly deal with problems associated with lighting conditions. When a photograph is taken in sunlight, an object has a different color on the resulting negative than when it is photographed under incandescent lighting. The photographer compensates for this effect by selecting film that is sensitive to the particular lighting conditions. The human determination of color, however, more or less compensates for this change in lighting. Colors appear more or less stable to us under differing light conditions.[8] Thus, our brains use information not only from the firing cones but also from the surrounding environment to make color determinations.

The appropriateness of a color also depends on the surrounding environment. Not only neighboring colors, but the size and purpose of the location in which the color appears help to determine whether it is suitable or not. Dark brown may be congenial in a bar, but is awkward in an infant's nursery. A small patch of a bright color, say pink, may liven up a room which would be made unbearable if the entire room were painted in that color. Sometimes a color is appropriate not because no better color can be found, but because it is neutral. That is, while a room may, for example, actually look best painted fuchsia—in terms of giving the feeling of space, of warmth, of light, and of comfort—we may nevertheless paint the room white because white is more in keeping with cultural norms. As long as white is appropriate, it need not be the "best" color in order to be chosen.[9]

Because of the complexity of the perception of color, there is no one scale of "colorfulness" on which to rank color; rather, in choosing color, whether for a room or for a canvas, we use a combination of skill, cultural sensitivity, a sense of balance, and intuition. The length AH in Figure 1, while perhaps useful in some contexts to help one make comparisons between colors, does not capture all that is important about color and thus fails to provide a reliable mechanism to help us choose which color is "best."

For much the same reasons that a color superscale cannot rank color, no value superscale can rank values. As was true of one's choice of color, a choice of which value is most important at the moment depends on, among other things, skill, cultural sensitivity, a sense of balance, and intuition. We choose our friendships, actions, and words in the context of our existing understanding of the world and in terms of the understanding we hope to achieve in the future.[10] That is, we choose not only to satisfy what we currently desire but to enable us to become what we wish to become. We study not necessarily for immediate pleasure but in order to become the type of person we hope to be. We care for our friends not only because they bring us immediate pleasure but because we want to be the type of person who values friendship. We may even choose to sacrifice our happiness or well-being in order to be someone that we hold in high regard;[11] we may give up our lives for a cause or for our people.[12]

Consider, for example, an individual, Gillian, choosing between returning to school to develop new skills in the hopes of finding a more fulfilling job and remaining in an unenjoyable, yet emotionally and financially stable job. The values militating in favor of returning to school are self-development, autonomy, and adventure; those against returning are stability, (financial) autonomy, and security. If there were a superscale of value, for example James Griffin's scale of well-being,[13] Gillian would be able to translate each of these values into some quotient of well-being and choose in accordance with the highest ranking value. Let us say that, in the particular case, Gillian chooses to return to school because she believes herself to be capable of greater things than her current job seems to permit. In the instant case, she ranks self-development ahead of stability and security on the superscale of well-being.[14]

While this example seems to support the contention that there exists a superscale on which one can rank values, when one examines Gillian's decision, one sees that the superscale actually played no role in her decision nor does it provide a useful guide as to which decisions Gillian is likely to make in the future.

The first thing to notice about Gillian's choice to go back to school is that she was only able to rank her values after she decided what she wanted to do. Intuitively, it is implausible to claim that, in her mental calculus, Gillian told herself that self-development would provide her with 50 points of well-being and that security would provide her with only 30 points and that, therefore, she should choose that option that most furthers self-development. What is intuitively more plausible is that Gillian examined who she understood herself to be, what she wanted to become, and what her values were at that moment—in other words, in the context of her entire framework of understanding—and made her decision on the basis of which choice appeared to further the goals she then had.[15] That is, Gillian only assigned points on the well-being scale after making her decision to go back to school; at that point, she understood herself to have ranked self-development ahead of security. The ranking of values on the scale of well-being was a result of Gillian having made her decision; it did not cause that decision to be made.

One may argue, though, that the ranking revealed through the example of Gillian's choice may provide a basis on which Gillian could rank values in the future. That is, Gillian's choice demonstrated her preferences, preferences that provide an understanding of which of Gillian's values are more important to her than others. But preferences based on revealed choices—choices made in particular contexts with particular understandings—fail to capture the essence of what is valuable.[16] Without the context and without the individual's understanding of the world, such revealed preferences tell us little about what is generally valuable; they only tell us what was valued in the particular circumstances of the decision.[17] One cannot extrapolate from such decisions to establish a value landscape. This is so because choices made need not be transitive—that is, simply because A was chosen over B and B was chosen over C does not imply that A would be chosen over C—[18] nor establish that what was chosen is better than that which was not.[19] Choices are made because they are thought good, not necessarily because they are thought to be better than the alternatives.[20]

The belief that values are commensurable, unless we are willing to accept a highly distorted view of values and of ourselves, is untenable. There is no reduction—whether to a single good, a single value, or a state of affairs—that can capture our understanding of the good.[21] It is not that commensurability offers an incomplete or unattainable deliberative process; it is that it offers merely a parody of such a process. In making choices, we constantly balance and enlarge our understanding of which goods are valuable and why they are so. Our languages and understanding of the world thus grow as individuals and societies attempt to balance the competing claims made upon them.

Leaving Out Nonmarket Values

Consider once again the dispute between the scientist wishing to conduct an autopsy on a cadaver in order to further her research and a religious believer who believes that cutting open a dead body is immoral. Each of these individuals values the body in different ways: the scientist in terms of increasing knowledge and the believer in terms of spirituality. Consider, moreover, that the cadaver is subject to property rights. Between the scientist and the believer, then, how ought a court to allocate such rights? The discourse applicable to this allocation is that of the market. According to market principles, one could argue that allocating property rights in the body to the scientist would encourage scientific research and, although not necessarily in the present case, increase the number of useful inventions made. These inventions would be traded on the market and increase well-being. Alternatively, one could argue that allocating property rights in the body to the scientist would stifle the research efforts of other researchers and thus discourage inventive activity overall.

It is much harder, however, to put the believer's way of valuing the body, as a sacred good, into the language of the market. One could try to argue that the believer would be likely to pay the most for the body in the market—in order to prevent autopsies—and, there-fore, in order to save transaction costs, we ought to allocate property rights in the cadaver to the believer. This argument fails, however, since we could not know *a priori* that the believer would, in fact, be willing to pay the most for the cadaver; only through the action of the market could this be established.

The disparate values of the scientist and of the believer do not translate equally, therefore, into the language of the market. While the believer could argue against the allocation of property rights to the scientist on market grounds—the stifling effect of monopolies—the believer cannot argue against this allocation in terms of the values that the believer holds in the cadaver. The scientist's position is some-what better. The scientist can rely on market arguments that reflect, at least in a significant way, the way the scientist values the cadaver: as a means of developing marketable inventions. But even some of the ways that the scientist values the cadaver may not be represented; for example, the scientist may value the cadaver for the pure joy of research or because the scientist is conducting the research out of respect for someone who died of the same disease as did the cadaver. These ways of valuing the body are not reflected in market discourse.

The Lack of Commensurability and Human Biological Materials

If, as argued, values are not commensurable, then subjecting human biological materials to property discourse may lead to the allocation of control over these materials without reference to significant noneconomic values inhering in them. Consider again the three examples set out at the end of chapter 7. In all three examples, market ways of viewing human biological materials existed side by side with such nonmarket values as community, identity, and altruism. The framework from which we understand human biological materials contains all these values, and each such value has a particular pull upon us.

In chapter 7 I discussed several values that were at stake in the decision in *Moore* v. *Regents of the University of California*.[22] These included not only the economic value of the cells in the cell line, but the values of dignity, autonomy, sharing and community, identity, and our understanding of health care. The majority in *Moore* based its decision on the perceived economic impact of its decision on research and development in the medical field. The court did not address, for example, whether the gains made in health care by this research were proportionate to the alienation patients may feel from an ever-more-technological and reductionalist approach to medicine exemplified by the research on Moore's cells.[23] While the majority in *Moore* did discuss Moore's autonomy, it did so only in the context of the decision to receive medical care—through the law of informed consent—and not in the context of giving Moore the choice to be altruistic in dedicating the cells to the community.

As discussed earlier, Golde's primary interest in Moore's spleen was a commercial one. This value easily translated into property discourse, premised as it was on market principles. On the other hand, the only value of Moore that translated into property discourse was his interest in receiving at least a share of the spleen's market value. While it is possible that this is truly the only interest that Moore had in his spleen, it would seem more plausible that it is just one of many ways that Moore valued his spleen. Moore may have felt, for example, that the commercial use of his body harmed his dignity; that is, the fact that someone had mined his body for valuable molecules may have felt disrespectful. Moore may have wanted to make a gift of his tissue by dedicating it to the public. This would have made him feel important and generous. Moore may have felt that permitting the research would increase his chances of survival and thus welcomed it. Moore may have felt that Golde's research might lead to a cure for cancer and thus help humanity.

While Moore may have felt any or all of these ways about his body, the values these feelings represent—dignity, charity, sharing, life, and community, among others—do not find voice within property discourse. This is because these values do not translate into the language of the market. Thus property rights are, and were in *Moore*, allocated without reference to them. As a result of the decision in *Moore*, Golde preserved his property rights to Moore's biological materials. Further, Golde's way of valuing these materials, in terms of their value on the market, prevailed.

Given that values are incommensurable, the values put aside by the *Moore* court will not be weighed and considered through market forces. The market has no mechanism by which to compare the values of autonomy, dignity, and increased health or to decide whether a holistic or a reductionalist approach to medicine is most beneficial. In fact, the very act of subjecting the cells to the market alters the ways in which they can be valued. The social meaning of Moore dedicating his cells to the community, for example, is different when those cells have a market value; Moore's gift becomes quantified.

Similarly, in the case of the ownership of fragments of cDNA, the public argument focused on whether research and development is best promoted by granting a monopoly or withholding it. By contrast, arguments about the nature of health care that are implicit in the decision whether to grant property rights in cDNA cannot be translated into a form that can be measured against these economic concerns. Whether the current technological approach to medicine is more or less likely to succeed than more holistic approaches is not something that can be determined through economic analysis. Nor can an economic analysis of cDNA reveal what effect granting property rights to them may have on our conceptions of identity or of the independence or personhood of those with certain genetic characteristics. Determining whether the fear that the geneticization of medicine may again lead to some form of eugenics[24] is real or imagined is a question of social, not economic, policy.

Conclusions about whether to grant property rights to cDNA and to whom these rights, if granted, ought to be allocated are likely to be wrong because only one factor, the economic impact of the decision on a certain type of medical research, counts. There are simply too many other ways of valuing cDNA within our frameworks but outside of the market for a conclusion made on this one basis to be correct.

The allocation of property rights to human organs may very well lead to an increase in the number of organs available for transplantation. This has an obvious salutary effect. But the negative impact of a decision to allocate such rights may be even more significant. Treating our bodies as chattels is qualitatively different from viewing them as sacred. The donation of blood to an unknown member of the community does not have the same social meaning as selling blood on the market. Taking some comfort from the thought that a child's death has helped another to live is vastly different from receiving a check because a child dies. Whether the ability to sell organs depreciates human life or dignity is a decision that ought not to be made on the basis of how much money a desperate individual is willing to pay.

Not only are the values inhering in human biological materials incommensurable, they are significantly transformed if they become property subject to trade on the market. Whether this transformation is good is hard to predict. What is certain is that the nature of the transformation is not considered when rights are allocated on the basis of economic value.

Subjecting human biological materials to the market fails to accord with the frameworks in which we understand and value these materials. Nonetheless, society must find ways of making decisions about these materials; the alternative is a series of *ad hoc* determinations about their control that may be more harmful to the values we cherish than would be a market analysis. The lack of commensurability is not an excuse not to attempt to arrive at a reasoned choice concerning control of human biological materials.

Making Comparisons without Commensurability

One way to make choices about human biological materials is to compare them. Simply because values are not commensurable does not imply that they are not comparable.[25] By comparable I mean that, in any given situation, we can discuss the claims made upon us by the various values that we hold. Within the particular circumstances of a decision, our values place concrete demands upon us. These demands interact, making some courses of action, or determinations of who we want to be, preferable to others. We can evaluate the force that each value has on us, taking into account the interaction between values, our goals, our perception of ourselves, and the facts underlying the decision. There is no need to place values on a common scale to undertake such deliberation; rather, values amplify or modulate each other within the specific deliberative context. It is this interaction between values that any attempt at commensurability ignores. By ignoring such interaction, commensurability fails to respond to the very real demands put upon us when we deliberate.

Consider again *Local 1330, United Steel Workers of America v. United States Steel Corp.*[26] Recall that, in that case, the parties were contesting control over two steel mills in Youngstown. The community and U.S. Steel valued the mills in dramatically different ways. The community valued the mills in terms of autonomy, community, and reliance; U.S. Steel valued the mills as a means to make a profit. Recall further that the *U.S. Steel* court held that, as much as it respected the ways in which the community valued the mills, there was no basis in law on which the court could further those values. That is, the only values that the court could directly consider were market values. The court found that its decision had to ensure that the mills were tradeable on the market so that mills in general would be put to their highest use.

Assume, however, that the *U.S. Steel* court had been convinced that the market was unable to ensure that the mills would be put to their highest use because the values inhering in the mills were incommensurable. The court would then have had only two choices: to allocate property rights only after examining and comparing the incommensurable values inhering in the mills, or to assign property rights based on market values alone but with the recognition that the law in a guise other than property would address the other nonmarket values inhering in mills. The choice of doing nothing—that is, not deciding who had property rights in the mills—would have been unacceptable; the court had to determine whether U.S. Steel could tear down the mills or whether the employees of U.S. Steel and the Youngstown community could run the mills.

If the *U.S. Steel* court had decided to undertake the admittedly arduous task of examining the various values inhering in the mills, it would have had to determine on what basis it was going to determine which values it would further and which values it would not. Further, because choices among values are contingent on the complete set of values held by the decision maker and require balance and subtlety, the court could strive at best to base its determination on certain of the values inhering in the mills that it believed were particularly important. But because of the contingencies and the impossibility of knowing what balance ought to be struck in other, even similar, cases, the court could not hope to articulate rules that would be applicable without substantive review in the future. In recognition of this, the court could seek to clearly articulate which values it attempted to further, the reasons why it chose those values, and what other important values were at stake. If the court clearly set out these points, future courts, having knowledge of whether the goals set out in the decision were actually achieved, holding a different mix of values, and having an appreciation of the subtleties of the case before them, could reevaluate the balance struck in the original decision in making their own decisions.

For example, imagine that the *U.S. Steel* court had held that, in its judgment, the value of community was strongly implicated in the mills. Shutting down the mills would lead to the loss of community for the thousands of residents of Youngstown. The court may have concluded that, given the great reliance that the people of Youngstown had developed over the years on the mills with the encouragement of U.S. Steel, the harm to community of shutting down the mills outweighed any theoretical loss to market values introduced through the allocation of property rights to members of the community. At the same time, the court would have had to discuss the nature of the loss to economic values that it anticipated: that, for example, third parties would be less interested in purchasing the mill because of uncertainty of title and that others would be less interested in investing in the construction of mills because of the possibility that they would lose control over the mill. Armed with such a decision, future courts could determine whether the *U.S. Steel* court was justified in its anticipation of the positive effects of its decision on the value of community and on the negative effects of its decision on economic values. This future court could then reevaluate the decision reached in *U.S. Steel*.

The second option available to the *U.S. Steel* court would be to make its property-law decision on the basis of furthering market values and leaving other areas of the law to address the other values inhering in the mills. This option will be discussed in the next chapter.

The *U.S. Steel* court had no option but to recognize some property right in the steel mills. After all, the mills have been treated as property by the courts, the legislature, and those running the mills for a long time. The court did not, as stated earlier, have the option of deciding that steel mills should not be property. That is, since steel mills have traditionally been subjected to property discourse, it would be extremely difficult to remove them from this discourse now.

The human body and human health have not, traditionally, been considered to be property. The option of concluding that these goods ought not to be subjected to property discourse is a real one. We can, as a society, conclude that the body and health are not and ought not to be property. If the body and health are not property, they will not be evaluated within a discourse that focuses on their market aspects rather than the nonmarket values inhering in them.

We have the opportunity to develop ways to treat cell lines, cDNA, and human organs that are sensitive to the many different ways that we value these human biological materials. We are not faced with the prospect of removing these goods from property discourse; rather, we can decide not to subject them to this discourse in the first place.

If the case of *Moore* were reconsidered outside of property discourse, the various values involved could be compared and balanced against one another. We would have to explicitly discuss the approach, reductionalist or holistic, that we are taking to health care. We would need to talk about the role of the patient in the health care process. We would have to address the issue of how tied individuals' identities are to their bodies or body components. We would have to turn our minds to the meaning of sharing in the context of life and health. If we make our assumptions and approaches explicit in our judgment, instead of hiding them behind the facade of market forces, a later decision maker could test them against reality and against the frameworks that exist at that time. We would not so much aim at getting the decision right—given the many values we could hold in our frameworks and their incommensurability, there is no right answer—but at making it understandable.

We could decide, for example, that neither Moore nor Golde owns the cell line, but that it belongs to some nonprofit nongovernmental organization, such as the Red Cross. That organization would be entitled to license the use of the cell line as it saw fit. We could provide representation of different segments of society on an ethics board to make these determinations. The board could, in addition, be given a mandate to pursue both research aimed at therapeutic uses of the cell line and research aimed at discovering the interaction between individuals and the environment on the incidence of disease. We could also give Moore some choice by allowing him to choose the organization that will control the cells. We can encourage Golde to conduct his research by ensuring that he will be granted a license to use the cell line in his research.

One could apply a similar approach to the sequences of cDNA fragments. These sequences could, for example, be placed on an electronic bulletin board. The proceeds from the downloading of these sequences could be used to fund other research, both the therapeutic and the holistic kind.

Instead of trying to increase the supply of transplantable organs by using market forces, we could use existing fora—such as schools, community centers, and religious institutions—to discuss the importance of community and the role sharing and altruism have in developing a sense of community. Such an approach, although requiring organization and patience, not only may increase the number of organs available, but may foster stronger communities.

No one formula for dealing with human biological materials is likely to emerge from this suggested approach. This is as it should be, since the values inhering in these materials take on different forms at different times, depending on the type of material being discussed.

One way to add this flexibility to property discourse is to supplement this discourse with other ways, within the law, of discussing human biological materials. Just as the majority in *Moore* supplemented its property-law analysis with a discussion of the law of informed consent, it may be possible to deal with the economic aspects of human biological materials within property discourse and deal with community values or autonomy through the law of charities or through human-rights legislation. This option will be discussed in the next chapter. As the discussion earlier in this chapter illustrates, however, once a good is subjected to market forces, the social meaning of that good may undergo such a transformation that we no longer value it in the same way.

In addition to the option of supplementing property law with other branches of the law, property discourse may, as discussed in the next chapter, change over time to permit a full discussion of the noneconomic values inhering in the goods subject to the discourse. Should such a change occur, we can then ask ourselves again whether to treat human biological materials as property. In the meantime, unless we can successfully supplement property discourse with other discourses, the best way to ensure that all of the values inhering in these materials are considered is to make decisions about them outside of property discourse.

This chapter illustrated that there are many values inhering in the human body and in health care that are not appropriately considered in property discourse, founded as it is on market values. This occurs for two reasons. First, because of the assumption that the market commensurates all values, courts confidently put aside consideration of nonmarket values in the expectation that the market will weigh these values indirectly. Second, the market fails to consider nonmarket values because the assumption that values are commensurable is incorrect. Together, these failures lead to the conclusion that property discourse, as currently practiced, is an inappropriate one for the determination of rights to human biological materials.

9

Unaccounted and Unaccountable Value

[N]ow I knew that the more the Dinosaurs disappear, the more they extend their dominion, and over forests far more vast than those that cover the continents: in the labyrinth of the survivors' thoughts. From the semidarkness of fears and doubts of now ignorant generations, the Dinosaurs continued to extend their necks, to raise their taloned hoofs, and when the last shadow of their image had been erased, their name went on, superimposed on all meanings, perpetuating their presence in relations among living beings. Now, when the name too had been erased, they would become one thing with the mute and anonymous molds of thought, through which thoughts take on form and substance: by the New Ones, and by those who would come after the New Ones, and those who would come even after them.[1]

Even when the law undergoes a seemingly pivotal change in one area, it takes many years before this change makes itself felt in other areas of the law and in society. The constitutional abolition of slavery in 1865,[2] for example, represented a fundamental change in property law. Yet, for all the importance of this change, it was not until the middle of this century that courts recognized the inherent inequality of social segregation[3] and another twenty years before the courts actively enforced desegregation.[4] Even now, a decade shy of the 150th anniversary of the abolition of slavery, the effects of slavery and the property regime that permitted it continue to dramatically shape American society.

The last chapters have illustrated that property discourse focuses on the economic values inhering in a good to the exclusion of the other values inhering in that good. This raises the concern that, if

164

human biological materials are made the subject matter of property rights, and hence property discourse, the legal system will allocate rights to those materials on the basis of furthering market values while ignoring the effects that these rights may have on other, noneconomic, values inhering in such material. This is what happened with respect to nonhuman biological materials in *Diamond v. Chakrabarty*.[5] The Court conducted its analysis in terms of market factors and deliberately refrained from examining nonmarket considerations such as safety, human health, and the value of life in deciding to accord Chakrabarty patent rights in the bacteria.[6]

Three routes can be taken in order to avoid establishing rights to human biological materials that ignore important nonmarket values inhering in such materials. First, we can reformulate property discourse to include a direct and open examination of these other values. Second, we can attempt to supplement property rights that are allocated on the basis of market considerations with rights based on other ways of valuing human biological materials.[7] Third, we can hold that human biological materials are not property and thus exempt them from property discourse. In the last case we would have to find some alternative way of dealing with these materials.

The capacity of property discourse to include or coexist with an explicit consideration of nonmarket values lies at the heart of our choice between these three strategies. If property discourse is open to change and this change can be brought about before property rights are fixed in human biological materials, then property law would be an appropriate vehicle through which to balance the many values inhering in these materials. If property law either is not open to such change or is open to change only over the long term, then property law alone will not adequately provide the opportunity to discuss all the values that inhere in human biological materials. The question then becomes whether property law ought to be a component of that discussion. As long as property discourse does not displace or trump other discourses, then we can consider the market aspects of a good through property discourse and other aspects of the good through other branches of the law. On the other hand, if property discourse has a tendency to displace other discourses—either because the role of property in law is such that property rights tend to trump other rights or because the substance of property discourse, market rhetoric, tends to discourage other discourses—then we ought not to discuss human biological materials within property discourse.

This chapter concludes the examination of property discourse as an appropriate way to discuss human biological materials by focusing on this discourse's capacity to include other discourses. By looking at the development and nature of contemporary property discourse, I conclude that, while this discourse has the capacity to change to include a direct consideration of noneconomic values, this change will not occur in the near future. Therefore, subjecting human biological materials to this discourse in the near future will result in the allocation of property rights in a manner that does not adequately consider noneconomic values. Further, because property rights are so fundamental in the law and because the nature of market rhetoric is to discourage direct consideration of noneconomic values, it is improbable, once human biological materials are made the subject of property rights, that other discourses would be able to correct for noneconomic aspects left out of property discourse's calculus. Therefore, given that human biological materials have not, except in fairly minor ways, been analyzed within property discourse, I conclude that such materials ought not now to be subjected to property rights.

Is Property Discourse Flexible?

As set out, the first option for dealing with property discourse's focus on market values is to open up the discourse to other competing, nonmarket, values. This would lead a court away from simply allocating property rights on the basis of factors such as whether a good can be traded on the market, whether certainty of title provides an economic motivation to create more of that good, and whether the granting of rights tends to hinder further development, and toward an allocation of property rights on the basis of a combination of these economic factors and such noneconomic values as human dignity, human health, environmental safety, and self-development.

Legal theorists have proposed a number of differing ways in which to expand property discourse. Margaret Jane Radin, for example, suggests that property rights ought to be created in order to promote self-development.[8] On her theory, drawn from Hegel,[9] individuals need to control portions of their environment so as to develop into free, responsible persons. An individual grows by investing his or her will in objects existing in the external world. Radin argues that property entitlements ought to be granted to individuals to encourage this process. According to her view, goods are important in various ways to one's self-development. Stronger property entitlements ought to be created to those goods with which we are most closely bound, such as heirlooms, wedding rings, and homes.[10] Weaker entitlements ought to be allocated to goods that we value only instrumentally, such as money and objects we mass-produce. This understanding of property encourages individuals to value goods intrinsically as embodiments of themselves and instrumentally as means to self-development.

William Simon argues that property ought to promote democracy and community involvement.[11] He suggests that property entitlements ought to be created in such a fashion that individuals are encouraged to view their property interests as stakes in the community rather than as a means for individual profit. This can be accomplished, according to Simon, by permitting individuals to transfer their property only to other members of the community and by placing limits on the quantity of goods that any one individual can hold. These constraints, Simon posits, provide individuals with material security and protection against subordination to either wealthy individuals or an impersonal market, and promote political responsibility. This understanding of property, therefore, promotes valuing goods as one's investment in the community and as providing one with a sense of place and commitment.

Laura Underkuffler's theory of property, which she calls the comprehensive approach, aims at promoting individual self-mastery.[12] On this view, property rights mediate between the interests of the individual and those of the collective, without preferring either absolutely. Underkuffler argues that property rights ought to be created in goods beyond physical objects and their analogs. She suggests that human rights, such as freedom of conscience, free use of facilities, and free choice of employment ought to be subject to property rights.[13] According to Underkuffler, increasing the scope of property rights leads away from the conception of property as being an absolute right to a conception of property as a right contingent on the community interest.[14] The comprehensive approach attempts, therefore, to promote self-mastery within and while maintaining collective interests. Like Radin's theory, this understanding of property encourages individuals to value goods as means to self-development. In addition, like social-republican property, the comprehensive approach promotes valuing goods as providing one with a place in the community.

Richard Posner offers a significantly different rationale for property entitlements.[15] He suggests that property rights ought to be created and allocated so as to maximize wealth. Accordingly, Posner submits that an absolute property right to a good ought to be created where transaction costs in that good are low. Where such costs are high, on the other hand, no or at most a conditional property right ought to be created. Moreover, to ensure an economically efficient result, Posner argues that property rights to goods ought to be allocated to those individuals who value them the most. Unlike the other theories of property we examined, Posner's understanding of property encourages individuals to value goods only instrumentally, as means to maximize their wealth.

According to each of these theorists, property regimes ought to promote particular ways of valuing goods. For example, a wedding ring ought to be valued, on Radin's conception of property, as a symbol of love and a shared life; on Simon's view of property, as a stake in a long-term relationship; on Underkuffler's understanding of property, as a symbol of a socially sanctioned relationship; and, on Posner's conception of property, as wealth.[16] Most of the theorists discussed recognize, however, that much of contemporary property discourse fails to value goods according to their favored dimension. Nevertheless, implicitly in their writing, these theorists are hopeful that this situation can change and, further, that such change can occur within current property discourse. That is, they believe that the current conception of property is sufficiently flexible to allow for the changes sought.

Languages and Concepts

The fact that many differing conceptions of property exist does not guarantee that we can reshape current property discourse, focused as it is on economic values, into one that invites discussion of all kinds of values, economic and otherwise. Property discourse may be so entrenched in the law and the rights that members of society expect that any reconceptualization, if possible at all, could only occur over an extended period of time. On the other hand, given the advances in and promises of biotechnology, human biological materials will increasingly be the subject of disputes. Therefore, if the current conception of property is not changed in the very near future, we risk allocating rights to human biological materials on the basis of an unchanged property discourse that ignores significant noneconomic values.

In order to determine whether property discourse is open to change and, if so, the expected time frame for such a change, one needs to understand the nature of legal conceptions—including how they are formed, how they shape legal doctrine, and how they are changed.[17]

We live in a world that is at once given—in the sense that others like us exist; that we drink, breathe, and become hungry; and that rocks, trees, and rivers exist—and one that we have created—for example, literature, cars, aesthetics, and sports. We create the world in that we shape not only the form and availability of what is given, but we give such material meaning—that is, we situate what is given in our system of beliefs.[18] Our ability to create goes one step further, however. By shaping what is given and by constructing meaning out of it, we shape who we are. In the words of Hannah Arendt, all things that enter into the human world "constantly condition their human makers."[19]

For example, although the need for food is a given condition of our existence, we create the meaning of hunger, of taste, and of sharing. These created "things" then condition us; we grow food so as not to go hungry, we develop skills in cooking food in response to our ability to distinguish taste, and we eat with others to create rituals of sharing. Out of the interaction of these conditions and others grow additional conditions: the food market, education, and friends and family. Conditions amass atop conditions until we who live under them are unable to conceive of the world without sweet and sour, companionship, or skill.

We shape, and are simultaneously shaped by, things both tangible, such as a chair or a book, and intangible, such as rest or study. Just as a chair determines the manner in which we eat, our understanding of friends and of family determines with whom we eat. The result of our shaping is that we come to understand the world not in its given form but in the form in which we have reshaped it; we only understand things within the framework[20]—the collection of values we hold and their orientation to one another—of understanding in which we have fixed them. Food is not simply bare sustenance; it is sweet or bitter, heavy or light, eaten alone, with family or with friends, it is satisfying or is lacking, it is prepared with care or indifference, and its consumption emphasizes contentment or loneliness.

As we reshape the given universe, we create needs and opportunities for ourselves. In reshaping food, we create the need for chefs and for developed palates on the one hand, and for famine relief and aid workers on the other. These roles shape our lives and contribute to the formation of our identities.[21] The chef develops an understanding of texture, of color, of sour and salt, of presentation, of atmosphere, of freshness, and of scent: an understanding beyond the experience of the rest of us. The aid worker comes to know of degrees of hunger, of disease, of hope and hopelessness, of stretching food as far as it can go, and of deciding who can benefit and who cannot. These understandings shape who we are and what we care about.

We do not reshape the given world merely by material instruments; we create meaning and roles from it through language, art, and action. Just as a spider builds its web to catch its prey and the beaver builds its dam to create a home, we create our world through words, images, and deeds.[22] Language provides the bridge between the world in its given form and the world as we understand it within our frameworks. "[L]anguages capture and drive our minds,"[23] simultaneously reshaping the givenness of the world and creating and altering who we are. Through words, images, and deeds, we create ourselves:

> We . . . are almost constantly engaged in presenting ourselves to others, and to ourselves, and hence *representing* ourselves— in language and gesture, external and internal. . . . Our human environment contains not just food and shelter, enemies to fight or flee, and conspecifics with whom to mate, but words, words, words. These words are potent elements of our environment that we readily incorporate, ingesting and extruding them, weaving them like spiderwebs into self-protective strings of *narrative*.[24]

Languages are not neutral factors in our understanding of the world. They open up vistas of thought while closing others off. To have one word for "snow" instead of many, as the Inuit have,[25] is to conceive of one's natural environment in a very different way. Similarly, to think of a family as a married man and woman with several children, as the traditional Western family is usually depicted, is far different from conceiving of a family as one or more parents of the same or different sex with or without children.[26] Thus, languages incorporate our ideologies, or ideology becomes reified in our language.[27]

To illustrate the effect that language has on our thought, consider the label "illness." While it appears ostensibly neutral, once this label is attached to some set of characteristics, it transforms the way we understand those characteristics. As Irving K. Zola explains:

> By the very acceptance of a specific behaviour as an illness and the definition of illness as an undesirable state the issue becomes not *whether* to deal with a particular problem but *how* and *when*. Thus, the debate over homosexuality, drugs, abortion, hyperactive children, antisocial behaviour, becomes focussed on the degree of sickness attached to the phenomenon in question (and its carriers) or the extent of *a* 'health' risk which *is* involved. And the more principled, more perplexing, or even moral issue of *what* freedom should an individual have over his/her body, or what else, besides the individual, needs treating is shunted aside.[28]

The confirmation hearings of Clarence Thomas as a justice on the United States Supreme Court several years ago exemplified the power of the label "illness."[29] At those hearings, Anita Hill testified that Thomas had sexually harassed her at work. Thomas supporters on the judiciary committee did not want to call Hill a liar, but still wanted to undermine her testimony. To the extent they succeeded, they did so by attaching the label "ill" to Hill. By making unsupported and, presumably, unsupportable psychological diagnoses of Hill, the Thomas supporters attempted to show that while Hill may have *believed* what she was saying, she only believed it because she was sick. Hill was thus depicted not as a liar but as sick and deluded. The senators, playing the part of doctors, were "neutrally" determining what was wrong with her. Since Hill was presumed to be "ill," what she had to say about her "illness" was taken as a symptom of the disease, not as rebuttal.[30]

The Language of the Market

As discussed throughout this book, the label "property" is closely wedded to market values. Each implies the other—material that promotes market values is labeled property and material that is labeled property is seen to promote market values. The power of the language of property must not be underestimated. As James Boyd White has pointed out, "When we speak our languages we cannot help believing them, we cannot help participating, emotionally and ethically and politically, in the worlds they create and in the structures of perception and feeling they offer us. In time the soldier wants to go to war."[31]

The language of the market prematurely ends discussion about other ways of valuing goods.[32] This language encourages the participant to understand and accept that the world functions according to "self-interest":

> [E]conomics cannot, in principle talk about any activity, any pleasure or motive or interest, other than the acquisitive or instrumental one that it universalizes. (Indeed it does not talk about this either but merely assumes and acts upon it.) This is not to be "value free," as its apologists claim, but to make aggressive self-interest the central, indeed the only, value, for it is the only one that can be talked about in these terms. To come at it the other way, it is to claim that all motives and interests can be talked about, at least for some purposes, as if they were selfish, quantifiable, and interchangeable; this is to erase all worlds of meaning except its own.[33]

To speak the language of property is to accept the modes of evaluation implicit in that language. It is to speak as if the primary values to be promoted are those of the market. When we realize that other ways of valuing goods are at stake, as in *U.S. Steel*, we do not have the language to speak them. To analyze the world in terms of property discourse is not to see the world in terms of relationships, in terms of personal development, or any other way of valuing goods. While it may be proper for some goods to be valued for their contribution to market values, not all goods ought properly be valued in this way or only in this way. To talk about the latter goods only in the language of the market, and this is what we do when we attach the label "property," is to miss much of what is important about them.[34]

The Evolution of the Property Concept

Labels and language are difficult and slow to change. The law represents a complex organization of concepts and principles.[35] Adjusting one impacts on the rest; often the influence of the rest undermines the adjustment. Because of the complexity of the legal system, usually only small changes can be made at a time. It takes many such small changes to change a principle and more time and changes to more principles to change a significant branch of the law. Just as the abolition of slavery did not immediately result in the equality of blacks and whites, a change to one area of law takes many years to affect another.

The concept of property as based on market values evolved over the past 200 years to its present form.[36] According to Morton Horwitz, this evolution was one from absolute dominion to the promotion of use and development.[37] The speed of change in the eighteenth and nineteenth centuries, measured over decades and taking over 100 years to accomplish, illustrates that a fundamental shift in conception is possible, but only over a long period of time. The legal theorists' goal of transforming property law to incorporate values of self-development, community, political responsibility, etc., is not one, therefore, that will easily or soon be achieved. The weight of history and of rhetoric is against a quick change. Further, as Jennifer Nedelsky notes, there is no sure victory at the end:

> The very strength of the tradition of property makes it in some ways a precarious base of innovation. When one chooses to use property, redefined, to provide new kinds of constitutional protection for rights of autonomy, participation, or material well-being, one runs the risk that temporary advances will fall back before a long and much narrower tradition.[38]

Since market values are at the center of property law discourse, we risk viewing all goods called "property" in a very limited fashion. While this may not be particularly troublesome when applied to many goods—those that our society has traditionally and appropriately valued primarily as market goods such as stocks, paper clips, and pens—it raises serious concern when applied to such goods as the human body. Viewing the body while wearing the blinders of contemporary property discourse may result in legal decisions that fail to adequately account for the noneconomic values inhering in the body. For example, the understanding generated by valuing the body as a resource to be mined and as an opportunity for profit may very well lead to the development of defective health care policies.

Present Conceptions; Future Hopes

I am not arguing, however, that change is impossible or undesirable. While the introduction of new ways of valuing goods within property discourse will make this discourse a more flexible tool in protecting important social interests, one cannot expect that such introduction will occur for some considerable time. One should, therefore, be cautious in formulating strategies to achieve reform. One should be especially careful about attempts to protect goods that previously were not considered property through property law. Although such goods presently do not get the protection offered by property rights, neither do we risk allocating them in a way that ignores important noneconomic values inhering in them.

Instead of attempting to protect new goods through property law, I suggest the better strategy is to first attempt to change the way we talk about those goods already subject to property rights. One could, as Radin suggests, evaluate the respective property interests of landlords and tenants in terms of personal development.[39] Alternatively, one could argue that the owner of a culturally significant work of art must make the work available to the public. Only after property law has expanded to truly permit a full and open discussion of nonmarket ways of valuing goods should reformers and theorists seek to subject new goods—such as the human body or health—to property analysis.

For example, I do not agree with Radin's view that women should have a property right in their reproductive abilities for purposes of surrogacy, even if restrictions are placed on that property right so that a woman cannot "rent" her womb on the market.[40] Given that market values are reified in contemporary property law discourse, thinking of women's reproductive abilities in the language of property presents the very real possibility that we will blind ourselves to other ways of valuing both women's bodies, women themselves, and children. For example, we may fail to adequately consider the effects on the development of a child born through surrogacy.

Considering a woman's reproductive capacities as a property right with restrictions on the sale of them, as Radin suggests, presents an additional danger. Placing such restrictions runs counter to economic values. The power to transfer property rights is a central tenet of property law[41] because of its link to the market. Given the importance of economic values within property discourse, any restriction on the power to transfer will be treated with some hostility. Over time, the pressure to allow the sale of surrogacy services may win the day. A woman's reproductive capacities would then become a commodity and be valued as such. This path from an inalienable property right to a fully transferable right is one that has already been traveled. The right of publicity, which is now fully transferable and descendible, is one example of such a journey:

> Only two decades ago a celebrity had no cause of action against an advertiser who imitated her voice. Until the 1970's any commercial value associated with celebrity was personal to the star and entered the public domain at death. As recently as the early 1950's celebrities could not assign the right to use their name and likeness. At the beginning of this century the law denied relief even to the living person whose name or likeness was the object of illicit appropriation.[42]

Other Branches of the Law

The defects of the language of the market as applied to the human body cannot be remedied through other discourses in other branches of the law. Property law has historically been and continues to be such a central feature of our legal system and the financial incentives established through this branch of the law are so strong that it is unlikely that other discourses can fill in what is left out in property discourse. The right to property is, after all, not only venerated in the common law and civil law, but enshrined in the United States Constitution.[43] Its influence within the law remains strong despite the passing years and changes in legal theory:

> Legal as well as political rhetoric implied that property rights gave effect to some preexisting natural phenomenon—whose concreteness gave an intuitive certainty and substance to the legal construct. Lawyers' and judges' daily work with the mutability, variety and multiplicity of property rights seemed (for at least 150 years) not to have shaken their sense that property rights were different from other legal entitlements and deserved a special and protected status.[44]

The difficulty with property discourse is that it preempts other discourses. The conception of property as having absolute dominion, although supplanted, continues to inform our understanding of how property rights interact with other rights. A person holding a proprietary interest in a good is entitled to do anything with respect to that interest unless doing so is specifically prohibited.[45] On the other hand, a person with a nonproprietary interest in the good is not entitled to do anything with that good unless specifically entitled. For example, in *Zacchini v. Scripps-Howard Broadcasting Co.*,[46] the United States Supreme Court held that Zacchini's proprietary interest in his cannonball performance was sufficient to prevent a television station from broadcasting the performance as part of its newscast, despite the argument that this abridged the station's freedom of speech.

Property rights are both positive, in that the holder of such rights is entitled to use and possess the good that is the subject matter of the rights as she or he chooses, and negative, in that the holder of such rights is entitled to prevent others from making use of the good.[47] Someone having a nonproprietary interest in the good generally has only the negative right to prevent another, the owner, from using the good in a manner detrimental to the nonproperty claimant's interest. Thus, an owner of a factory can use the factory to manufacture goods, can demolish the factory, and can prevent others from entering into the factory. A neighbor of the factory has only the right to prevent certain uses of the factory such as using the factory in a way that pollutes.

The right to prevent certain activity is not always sufficient, however, for those valuing the human body in terms of noneconomic values. While the ability to prevent certain research could be vindicated through means other than property rights, the right to direct, to share in the benefits, and to publish results of research conducted on human biological materials cannot, for example, be vindicated without the rights of possession and of use. These rights are attributes of property. Thus, unless we can discuss the noneconomic values inhering in the body at the time property decisions are being made, we cannot fully vindicate these values.

Human Biological Materials as Nonproprietary Goods

Given the likelihood that property discourse will not soon evolve to encourage discussion of noneconomic values and given that property discourse preempts other discourses that do not focus exclusively on economic values, it is advisable not to discuss human biological materials, in which many noneconomic values inhere, in terms of property. That is, property discourse is an inappropriate forum for the discussion of how the law ought to regulate the new biotechnologies and reproductive technologies as applied to the human body.

In *Moore v. Regents of the University of California*,[48] while both Justice Mosk and Justice Arabian wished to safeguard certain noneconomic values inhering in the human body, only Justice Arabian's suggestion that the body not be discussed within property discourse offers any possibility that this wish can be fulfilled. While Radin, Simon, Underkuffler, and Justice Mosk are likely correct that property law could have developed in such a fashion as to value goods, including the human body, in terms of self-development, community, self-mastery, or dignity, property law did not develop in this way.[49] The human body, which has largely escaped discussion within property law, ought not now to be treated as property.

New Directions

Rejecting property-law analysis for the human body does not end the inquiry into how the law ought to respond to the very real and practical needs of the biotechnology industry. The *status quo*, in which researchers and pharmaceutical companies are likely to be able to apply for and receive patent rights in human tissues while the sources of these tissues are left without compensation, is not acceptable. In such a situation, the human body continues to be discussed in market terms, given that human genes and cells are still patentable. Patients will continue to feel exploited as their bodies are treated as natural resources by others while they are not permitted to participate in this exploitation. In order to adequately respond to the needs of patients, researchers, pharmaceutical companies, and the public at large, a comprehensive, statutory scheme must be devised to regulate the rights and duties of the various participants. Such a scheme would have to be sufficiently flexible to permit discussion of various economic and noneconomic values. In addition, to prevent any attempt to introduce property discourse into the discussion of the human body, such a scheme would have to clearly exclude the application of property law, including patent law, to human biological materials.

Notes

CHAPTER 1 NOTES

1. W.E.B. Du Bois, *The Souls of Black Folks*, Signet Books (New York: Penguin Books, 1982), p. 126.

2. Biotechnology has been defined as follows:

> **Biotechnology,** broadly defined, includes any technique that uses living organisms (or parts of organisms) to make or modify products, to improve plants or animals, or to develop micro-organisms for specific uses—including recently developed techniques such as gene cloning and cell fusion.

U.S. Congress, Office of Technology Assessment, *New Developments in Biotechnology: Ownership of Human Tissues and Cells—Special Report* (Washington, D.C.: U.S. Congress, Office of Technology Assessment, 1987), p. 24. It should be noted that, according to this definition, the effort to sequence the human genome is, itself, a biotechnology.

3. Deoxyribonucleic acid (DNA) contains the genetic material for most life forms.

4. The application of property law to human biological materials caused a transatlantic skirmish over whether the National Institutes of Health (NIH) ought to apply for and be granted patent rights over relatively short sequences of human DNA. See Leslie Roberts, "Genome Patent Fight Erupts," *Science* 254 (1991): 184; Gina Kolata, "Biologist's Speedy Gene Method Scares Peers but Gains Backer," *New York Times*, 28 July 1992, p. 5(B); Rebecca S. Eisenberg, "Genes, Patents, and Product Development," *Science* 257 (1992): 903; Reid G. Adler, "Genome Research: Fulfilling the Public's Expectations for Knowledge and Commercialization," *Science* 257 (1992): 908; Thomas D. Kiley, "Patents on Random Complementary DNA Fragments?," *Science* 257 (1992): 915; Gina Kolata, "In Rush to Patent Genes, the Claims Get Smaller," *New York Times*, 6 September 1992, sec. 4, p. 12; Leslie Roberts, "Rumors Fly Over Rejection of NIH Claim," *Science* 257 (1992): 1855; Leslie Roberts, "Top HHS Lawyer Seeks to Block NIH," *Science* 258 (1992): 209; Christopher Anderson, "NIH to Appeal Patent Decision," *Science* 259 (1993): 302; Christopher Anderson, "NIH Drops Bid for Gene Patents," *Science* 263 (1994): 909.

Disputes have also arisen with respect to public access to DNA databases. See Eliot Marshall, "HGS Opens Its Databanks—For A Price," *Science* 266 (1994): 25; Eliot Marshall, "A Showdown Over Gene Fragments," *Science* 266 (1994): 208.

5. The Office of Technology Assessment defines human biological materials as follows:

> What are **human biological materials**? Human bodies contain a number of parts that can be useful in biomedical research. Healthy individuals continually produce a number of replenishable substances, including blood, skin, bone marrow, hair, urine, perspiration, saliva, milk, semen, and tears. Human bodies also contain nonreplenishing parts, such as oocytes or organs, which may either be vital (e.g., heart) or to some extent expendable (e.g., lymph nodes or a second kidney). Finally, diseased examples of these body parts also exist.

Office of Technology Assessment, *Ownership of Human Tissues and Cells*, p. 24. Unlike the Office of Technology Assessment, which distinguishes undeveloped human biological materials from biological inventions developed from such materials, ibid., in this book I include, unless I state otherwise, both undeveloped and developed materials within the definition of human biological materials. I do this because certain substances, for example hormones, are the developed products of biotechnological research yet identical, except with respect to purity, to naturally occurring substances.

6. See, generally, Morton J. Horwitz, *The Transformation of American Law 1780–1860* (Cambridge, Mass.: Harvard University Press, 1977).

7. The system of property generally led to men holding title to land.

8. A.M. Honoré, "Ownership," in *Oxford Essays in Jurisprudence*, ed. A.G. Guest (London: Oxford University Press, 1961), p. 113.

9. I discuss this in more detail in Richard Gold, "A Structural Dynamic Theory of Law," *Queen's Law Journal* 16 (1991): 347.

10. Elizabeth Anderson, *Value in Ethics and Economics* (Cambridge, Mass.: Harvard University Press, 1993), pp. 4 and 12.

11. Michael Walzer, *Spheres of Justice: A Defense of Pluralism and Equality* (New York: Basic Books, 1983), pp. 86–91. The right to health care has been recognized internationally, in human rights instruments; see, e.g., Organization of American States, *Additional Protocol to the American Convention of Human Rights in the Area of Economic, Social and Cultural Rights*, Article 10 (1988), and through the provision of state health care in most Western countries; see, e.g., Milton I. Roemer, *National Health Systems of the World* (New York: Oxford University Press, 1991).

CHAPTER 2 NOTES

1. William A. Ewing, *The Body: Photographs of the Human Form* (San Francisco: Chronicle Books, 1994), pp. 9–10.

2. 2005 is the goal set for the completion of the Human Genome Project, an international effort to map the genome. See Christopher Wills, *Exons, Introns, and Talking Genes* (U.S.A.: Basic Books, 1991), p.10. Wills defines genome as "[a]ll the genes of an organism, along with all the other DNA of the chromosomes." Ibid., p. 345.

3. For an overview of these technologies, see generally Robert Shapiro, *The Human Blueprint: The Race to Unlock the Secrets of Our Genetic Code* (New York: Bantam Books, 1991), passim; Wills, *Exons, Introns, and Talking Genes*, passim. Gene therapy involves the addition of genetic material to a patient's cells in order to alleviate the symptoms of a genetic disease. Wills, *Exons, Introns, and Talking Genes*, p. 344.

4. In fact, human health care is the focus of most research and development in the biotechnology industry generally. U.S. Congress, Office of Technology Assessment, *New Developments in Biotechnology: U.S. Investment—Summary* (Washington, D.C.: U.S. Congress, Office of Technology Assessment, 1988), p. 3. Approximately half of all researchers in the health field use human tissues. Office of Technology Assessment, *Ownership of Human Tissues and Cells*, p. 52.

5. Lawrence K. Altman, "Vaccine Offers Hope in Cancer Cases," *New York Times*, 22 October 1992, p. 8(A).

6. See, e.g., Richard C. Mulligan, "The Basic Science of Gene Therapy," *Science* 260 (1993): 926; Natalie Angier, "U.S. Permits Use of Genes in Treating Cystic Fibrosis," *New York Times*, 4 December 1992, p. 11(A); see generally Wills, *Exons, Introns, and Talking Genes*.

7. 51 Cal. 3d 120 (1990). The facts as outlined in the text are set out in *Moore* at 125–28.

8. Moore did so at his own expense.

9. See Office of Technology Assessment, *Ownership of Human Tissues and Cells*, p. 35.

10. Ibid., 32–34.

11. This estimate, based on the value of the cell line and other products until 1990, was provided by Moore in his complaint. Moore v. Regents of the Univ. of Cal., 51 Cal. 3d at 127.

12. Moore v. Regents of Univ. of Cal., 249 Cal. Rptr. 494 (Ct. App. 1988).

13. Moore v. Regents of Univ. of Cal., 51 Cal. 3d 120, 134–47 (1990).

14. Ibid., 128–34.

15. There has been a plethora of academic articles discussing *Moore* and the issues it raises. See, e.g., Lori B. Andrews, "My Body My Property," *Hastings Center Report* 16, no. 5 (1986): 28; Michelle B. Bray, Note, "Personalizing Personalty: Toward a Property Right in Human Bodies," *Texas Law Review* 69, (1990): 209; Mary T. Danforth, "Cells, Sales and Royalties: The Patient's Right to a Portion of the Profits," *Yale Law and Policy Review* 6 (1988): 179; Roy Hardiman, "Toward the Right of Commerciality: Recognizing Property Rights in the Commercial Value of Human Tissue," *UCLA Law Review* 34 (1986): 207; Christopher Hayer, "Moore v. Regents of University of California: The Right of Property in Human Tissue and Its Effect on Medical Research," *Rutgers Computer and Technology Law Journal* 16 (1990): 629; Laura M. Ivey, Note, "Moore v. Regents of the University of California: Insufficient Protection of Patients' Rights in the Biotechnological Market," *Georgia Law Review* 25 (1991):

489; Patricia A. Martin and Martin L. Lagod, "Biotechnology and the Commercial Use of Human Cells: Toward an Organic View of Life and Technology," *Santa Clara Computer and High Technology Law Journal* 5 (1989): 211; Randy W. Marusyk and Margaret S. Swain, "A Question of Property Rights in the Human Body," *Ottawa Law Review* 21 (1989): 351; Patricia M. Parker, "Recognizing Property Interests in Bodily Tissues: A Need for Legislative Guidance," *Journal of Legal Medicine* 10 (1989): 357; Russell Scott, *The Body as Property* (New York: Viking Press, 1981).

16. Moore v. Regents of the Univ. of Cal., 51 Cal. 3d 120 at 146.

17. Ibid., quoting Office of Technology Assessment, *Ownership of Human Tissues and Cells*, p. 27.

18. In reaching this conclusion, the majority referred to some of the anticipated negative effects of holding that patients have a property right in their tissues:

> The extension of conversion law into this area will hinder research by restricting access to the necessary raw materials. Thousands of human cell lines already exist in tissue repositories . . . These repositories respond to tens of thousands of requests for samples annually. . . At present, human cell lines are routinely copied and distributed to other researchers for experimental purposes, usually free of charge. This exchange of scientific materials, which still is relatively free and efficient, will surely be compromised if each cell sample becomes the potential subject matter of a lawsuit.

Moore v. Regents of the Univ. of Cal., 51 Cal. 3d at 144–45.

19. Ibid., 143.

20. The majority stated that other ways of valuing the body ought to be protected outside the law of property, for example, by the law of informed consent:

> Yet one may earnestly wish to protect privacy and dignity without accepting the extremely problematic conclusion that interference with those interests amounts to a conversion of personal property. Nor is it necessary to force the round pegs of "privacy" and "dignity" into the square hole of "property" in order to protect the patient, since the fiduciary-duty and informed-consent theories protect these interests directly by requiring full disclosure.

Moore v. Regents of the Univ. of Cal., 51 Cal. 3d at 140.

21. See Robert G. Evans, *Strained Mercy: The Economics of Canadian Health Care* (Toronto: Butterworths, 1984), pp. 71–73; G.M. Ginsberg, "Cost-Effectiveness Analysis, Cost-Benefit Analysis and the Value of Life in Health Care and Prevention," in *Costs and Benefits in Health Care and Prevention: An International Approach to Priorities in Medicine*, ed. U. Laaser et al. (Berlin: Springer-Verlag, 1990), pp. 6–7.

22. Justice Broussard wrote that "the majority's rejection of plaintiff's conversion cause of action does *not* mean that body parts may not be bought or sold for research or commercial purposes or that *no* private individual or entity may benefit economically from the fortuitous value of plaintiff's diseased cells." Moore v. Regents of the Univ. of Cal., 51 Cal. 3d at 160 (Broussard, J., concurring in part and dissenting in part).

23. Justice Broussard criticized the majority for failing to address patients' interests in such material. "[T]he opinion speaks only of the 'patient's right to make autonomous medical decisions' and fails even to mention the patient's interest in obtaining the economic value, if any, that may adhere in the subsequent use of his own body parts." Ibid., 159.

24. Ibid., 154–55, 158–59.

25. He held:

Thus, the majority's analysis cannot rest on the broad proposition that a removed body part is not property, but rather rests on the proposition that *a patient* retains no ownership interest in a body part once the body part has been removed from his or her body.

Ibid., 153–54.

26. Ibid., 160. See also ibid, 159.

27. See, e.g., the following statement by Justice Broussard:

It is certainly arguable that, as a matter of policy or morality, it would be wiser to prohibit any private individual or entity from profiting from the fortuitous value that adheres in a part of a human body, and instead to require all valuable excised body parts to be deposited in a public repository which would make such materials freely available to all scientists for the betterment of society as a whole. The Legislature, if it wished, could create such a system, as it has done with respect to organs that are donated for transplantation. To date, however, the Legislature has not adopted such a system for organs that are to be used for research or commercial purposes.

Ibid., 172.

28. Justice Mosk identified two noneconomic values implicated in the decision of whether to grant Moore a property right in his own tissues. These two values, dignity and equity, Justice Mosk held, trumped the majority's market concerns not because of their greater price, but because they exist outside of the market, on the moral plane. See Moore v. Regents of the Univ of Cal., 51 Cal. 3d at 173–77 (Mosk, J., dissenting).

29. Justice Mosk argued, elsewhere in his opinion, that the majority's market analysis is wrong on the facts in *Moore*. Ibid., 170–73.

30. Ibid., 175, 178–82.

31. Anderson, *Value in Ethics and Economics*, 44–64; Martha C. Nussbaum, *The Fragility of Goodness: Luck and Ethics in Greek Tragedy and Philosophy* (Cambridge, Engl.: Cambridge University Press, 1986), p. 310; Charles Taylor,

Sources of the Self: The Making of the Modern Identity (Cambridge, Mass.: Harvard University Press, 1989), pp. 77–79.

32. See generally, Evans, *Strained Mercy*, pp. 71–73, 75–76; Ginsberg, "Cost-Effectiveness Analysis," pp. 6–7; Ethan A. Halm and Annetine C. Gelijns, "An Introduction to the Changing Economics of Technological Innovation in Medicine," in *The Changing Economics of Medical Technology*, ed. Annetine C. Gelijns and Ethan A. Halm (Washington, D.C.: National Academy Press, 1991), pp. 3–4.

33. Halm and Gelijns, "Introduction to Changing Economics," pp. 3–4.

34. Evans, *Strained Mercy*, p. 54; Ginsberg, "Cost-Effectiveness Analysis," pp. 6–7.

35. Evans, *Strained Mercy*, p. 93.

36. For example, does good health include absence of psychological stress and, if so, what kinds of stress? Does a broken heart constitute pain?

37. Ibid., 252–55.

38. Evans, *Strained Mercy*, 255–57; H.P. Galler, "The Willingness-To-Pay Approach: Caveats to Biased Application," in *Costs and Benefits in Health and Prevention: An International Approach to Priorities in Medicine*, ed. U. Laaser et al. (Berlin: Springer-Verlag, 1990), pp. 37–39.

39. Evans, *Strained Mercy*, pp. 263–64.

40. Ibid.

41. See Elaine Scarry, *The Body in Pain: The Making and Unmaking of the World* (New York: Oxford University Press, 1985).

42. Moore v. Regents of the Univ. of Cal., 51 Cal. 3d 120, 183 (1990).

43. "I write separately to give voice to a concern that I believe informs much of [the majority] opinion but finds little or no expression therein. I speak of the moral issue." Moore v. Regents of the Univ of Cal., 51 Cal. 3d at 148 (Arabian, J., concurring).

44. Ibid.

45. Justice Arabian's uncertainty about judicial competence is expressed throughout his opinion, for example:

> It is true, that this court has not often been deterred from deciding difficult legal issues simply because they require a choice between competing social or economic policies. The difference here, however, lies in the nature of the conflicting moral, philosophical and even religious values at stake, and in the profound implication of the position urged.

Ibid., 149.

46. In inviting the legislature to intervene, the majority did not contend that the legislature was better able to balance the myriad values at stake in *Moore*; rather, the majority argued that the legislature's superior access to empirical facts permitted the legislature to better evaluate the economic consequences of granting Moore a property right in his own tissue:

> If the scientific users of human cells are to be held liable for failing to investigate the consensual pedigree of their raw materials, we believe

the Legislature should make that decision. Complex policy choices affecting all society are involved, and "[l]egislatures, in making such policy decisions, have the ability to gather empirical evidence, solicit the advice of experts, and hold hearings at which all interested parties present evidence and express their views . . ." Legislative competence to act in this area is demonstrated by the existing statutes governing the use and disposition of human biological materials. Legislative interest is demonstrated by the extensive study recently commissioned by the United States Congress. Commentators are also recommending legislative solutions.

Moore v. Regents of the Univ. of Cal., 51 Cal. 3d at 147.

47. Justice Broussard's position on judicial competence is more ambiguous than that of the majority. He argued that the legislature may be better able than the courts to balance the values inhering in human biological materials. Moore v. Regents of the Univ of Cal., 51 Cal. 3d at 159. Justice Broussard nevertheless held that the court was competent to allocate property rights on the basis of market considerations.

Justice Mosk found, for his part, that there was no competency problem involved in *Moore.* Ibid., 163.

48. Moore v. Regents of the Univ. of Cal, 51 Cal. 3d at 149.

49. Justice Arabian's concern about judicial competency plays an important role in his belief that property discourse, as carried out in the courts, cannot accommodate nonmarket values:

> Does it uplift or degrade the "unique human persona" to treat human tissue as a fungible article of commerce? Would it advance or impede the human condition, spiritually or scientifically, by delivering the majestic force of the law behind plaintiff's claim? I do not know the answers to these troubling questions, nor am I willing—like Justice Mosk—to treat them simply as issues of "tort" law, susceptible of *judicial* resolution.

Ibid.

50. Ibid., 149.

51. Justice Arabian's conclusion is similar to that reached by Richard Titmuss, who has argued that a market in blood is incompatible with some community values such as altruism and social responsibility. Richard Titmuss, *The Gift Relationship: From Human Blood to Social Policy* (New York: Pantheon Books, 1971). Contra Eric Mack, "Dominos and the Fear of Commodification," in *NOMOS XXXI: Markets and Justice*, ed. John W. Chapman and J. Roland Pennock (New York: New York University Press, 1989), p. 217. Titmuss asserted that a market in goods such as human blood drives out the feeling that one is responsible for one's neighbor:

> By contrast, one of the functions of atomistic private market systems is to "free" men [and women] from any sense of obligation to or for other men [and women] regardless of the consequences to others who

cannot reciprocate, and to release some men [and women] (who are eligible to give) from a sense of inclusion in society at the cost of excluding other men [and women] (who are not eligible to give).

Titmuss, *The Gift Relationship*, p. 239. When one sees the poor lining up to sell blood, Titmuss argued, one feels released from the obligation to give blood for the benefit of others. When blood is bought and sold, we come to look on it as any other commodity. Ibid., 171. No longer is a blood donation an expression of trust that strangers will come to our aid, as we have come to theirs, when the need arises, *ibid.* at 238–39; rather, we come to trust the market to provide us with blood.

52. James Boyd White argues that such a discourse, based on market concerns, colonizes other concerns, reducing them to a single value, self-interest. James B. White, *Justice as Translation: An Essay in Cultural and Legal Criticism* (Chicago: University of Chicago Press, 1990), pp. 57–58.

53. See generally John Ratcliffe et al., "Perspectives on Prevention: Health Promotion vs. Health Protection," in *The End of an Illusion: The Future of Health Policy in Western Industrialized Nations*, ed. Jean de Kervasdoué, John R. Kimberly, and Victor G. Rodwin (Berkeley: University of California Press, 1984), p. 66.

54. Ibid., 66, 68–69. It is generally accepted among health policy analysts that health status and life expectancy are best promoted by social factors such as good sanitation, nutrition, housing, and education. Ibid.; Evans, *Strained Mercy*, p. 3; see also R.C. Lewontin, *Biology as Ideology: The Doctrine of DNA* (New York: HarperCollins, 1991), pp. 44–45; Ruth Hubbard and Elijah Wald, *Exploding the Gene Myth: How Genetic Information Is Produced and Manipulated by Scientists, Physicians, Employers, Insurance Companies, Educators, and Law Enforcers* (Boston: Beacon Press, 1993), p. 60; Karen Wright, "Going by the Numbers," *New York Times Magazine*, 15 December 1991, 58.

55. Robert G. Evans pointed to the paradox that relying on each individual health consumer to maximize his or her well-being produces an expensive and ineffective health care system:

> Suppose a group of people, a society, make their allocations between (efficacious) prevention and cure on the basis of individual marginal rates of substitution. By spending less on prevention, and more on cure, they may as a group have both shorter life expectancies *and* higher expenditure on life-prolonging care. (Any parallel with United States health care is accidental, though the micro-rationality argument does come from the United States.)

Evans, *Strained Mercy*, p. 256.

56. Abby Lippman has called this policy the "geneticization" of health care:

> Geneticization refers to an ongoing process by which differences between individuals are reduced to their DNA codes, with most disor-

ders, behaviors and physiological variations defined, at least in part, as genetic in origin. It refers as well to the process by which interventions employing genetic technologies are adopted to manage problems of health. Through this process, human biology is incorrectly equated with human genetics, implying that the latter acts alone to make us each the organism she or he is.

Abby Lippman, "Prenatal Genetic Testing and Screening: Constructing Needs and Reinforcing Inequities," *American Journal of Law and Medicine* 17 (1991): 17. See also Hubbard & Wald, *Exploding the Gene Myth*, pp. 5, 69.

Some recent developments support the claim that health care is becoming geneticized. See, e.g., Robert Wright, "The Evolution of Despair," *Time*, 28 August 1995, 32; Rachel Nowak, "Genetic Testing Set for Takeoff," *Science* 265 (1994): 464; Henry Hess, "How the mating game evolved," *(Toronto) Globe and Mail*, 6 July 1994, p. 12(A); David Ankney, "What if violent types are born, not made?," *(Toronto) Globe and Mail*, 6 July 1994, p. 20(A); Thomas J. Bouchard Jr., "Genes, Environment, and Personality," *Science* 264 (1994): 1700; "Genetic signposts on the road to cancer," *(Toronto) Globe and Mail*, 11 June 1994, p. 8(D); "Gene Linked for First Time to High Blood Pressure Risk," *New York Times*, 2 October 1992, p. 14(A); Gina Kolata, "Genetic Defects Detected in Embryos Just Days Old," *New York Times*, 24 September 1992, p. 1(A).

57. See, e.g., Lippman, "Prenatal Genetic Testing and Screening"; Ivan Illich, *Limits to Medicine: Medical Nemesis: The Expropriation of Health* (London: Penguin Books, 1976); Irving K. Zola, "Healthism and Disabling Medicalization," in *Disabling Professions*, ed. Ivan Illich et al. (London, Engl.: Marion Boyars, 1977), p. 41.

58. See Lippman, "Prenatal Genetic Testing and Screening", p. 17.

CHAPTER 3 NOTES

1. Alexis de Tocqueville, *Democracy in America*, ed. Phillips Bradley, Vintage Books (New York: Random House, [1840]), 2:268–69.

2. While the principal goal of the Human Genome Project is to map the entire human genome, along the way researchers will map the genomes of several other organisms including the bacterium, *Escherichia coli*, the best known variety of yeast, *Saccharomyces cerevisiae*, the nematode, the fruit fly, the mouse, and a plant. See Shapiro, *The Human Blueprint*, 263–65.

3. Christopher Anderson, "Genome Project Goes Commercial," *Science* 259 (1993): 300. See, e.g., Ann Gibbons, "Scripps Signs a Deal with Sandoz," *Science* 258 (1992): 1570; Christopher Anderson, "Scripps–Sandoz Deal Comes Under Fire," *Science* 259 (1993): 889; Christopher Anderson, "Scripps Backs Down on Controversial Sandoz Deal," *Science* 260 (1993): 1872; Christopher Anderson, "Scripps to Get Less From Sandoz," *Science* 264 (1994): 1077; see, generally, Marcia Barinaga, "Confusion on the Cutting Edge," *Science* 257 (1992): 616; Christopher Anderson, "Hughes' Tough Stand on Industry Ties," *Science* 259 (1993): 884.

4. Anderson, "Genome Project Goes Commercial," 300–01; Elizabeth Culotta, "New Startups Move in As Gene Therapy Goes Commercial," *Science* 260 (1993): 914.

5. One industry observer estimated that private investors have contributed approximately $300 million per year to biotechnology firms since 1987. Richard Stone, "Biotech Sails Into Heavy Financial Seas," *Science* 260 (1993): 908.

6. Anderson, "Genome Project Goes Commercial," 300.

7. This change in the role of researchers has occurred over the last dozen or so years:

> Ten years ago, it was unusual for a basic researcher in biology to have large holdings in a company directly related to his or her field of research. Today, in some fields it's hard to find a researcher who doesn't consult with or have equity in a hot biotech startup.

Barinaga, "Confusion on the Cutting Edge," 616. See also Hubbard & Wald, *Exploding the Gene Myth*, 2.

8. See, generally, Barinaga, "Confusion on the Cutting Edge," 616.

9. See, e.g., Hubbard and Wald, *Exploding the Gene Myth*, 119; Peter Aldhous, "French Gene Mappers at Crossroads," *Science* 263 (1994): 1552.

10. See, e.g., Gibbons, "Scripps Signs a Deal," 1570; Anderson, "Scripps–Sandoz Deal Comes Under Fire," 889.

11. See Hubbard & Wald, Exploding the Gene Myth, 121.

12. See, generally, Rebecca S. Eisenberg, "Patenting the Human Genome," *Emory Law Journal* 39 (1990): 740–44.

13. Individual responsibility in the sense that individuals are responsible for taking steps to prevent illness, such as staying away from toxic chemicals, rather than society being responsible for ensuring to such individuals an environment in which they are unlikely to be exposed to toxic chemicals. E.g., Dorothy Nelkin, "The Social Power of Genetic Information," in *The Code of Codes: Scientific and Social Issues in the Human Genome Project*, ed. Daniel J. Kevles and Leroy Hood (Cambridge, Mass.: Harvard University Press, 1992), pp. 183–89; Hubbard & Wald, *Exploding the Gene Myth*, 5; Lewontin, *Biology as Ideology*, 76–77; Zola, "Healthism and Disabling Medicalization," 62.

14. Dorothy Nelkin described the appeal to institutions, such as schools, of tests that take the blame for illness off society:

> Tests can be used to redefine socially derived syndromes as problems of the individual, placing blame in ways that reduce public accountability and protect routine institutional practices. The availability of biological tests, in effect, gives an organization a scientific means to deal with failures or unusual problems without threatening its basic values or disrupting its existing programs.

Nelkin, "Social Power of Genetic Information," 183. See also Evelyn F. Keller, "Nature, Nurture, and the Human Genome Project," in *The Code of Codes:*

Scientific and Social Issues in the Human Genome Project, ed. Daniel J. Kevles and Leroy Hood (Cambridge, Mass.: Harvard University Press, 1992), p. 281.

15. 51 Cal. 3d 120 (1990).

16. See, e.g., Honoré, "Ownership," 107; Kenneth J. Vandevelde, "The New Property of the Nineteenth Century: The Development of the Modern Concept of Property," *Buffalo Law Review* 29 (1980): 364; Arnold S. Weinrib, "Information and Property," *University of Toronto Law Journal* 38 (1988): 120.

17. The academic literature, while interesting, is less concerned with mapping out how the law is being applied under current conceptions of property than with how the law ought to be applied, assuming some ideal conception of property. I deal further with the academic literature in chapter 9.

18. I borrow this example from Margaret J. Radin, "Property and Personhood," *Stanford Law Review* 34 (1982): 959.

19. In fact, the jeweler may take more pride in the ring knowing that the wearer sincerely cherishes it than if the ring remained in the jeweler's possession.

20. From the point of view of market analysis, the highest use for a good is exactly that use to which the good would be put in a perfect market.

21. 51 Cal. 3d 120 (1990).

22. This argument was raised in the post-*Moore* case, Miles, Inc. v. Scripps Clinic and Research Found., 810 F.Supp. 1010, 1098 (S.D. Cal. 1993).

23. *See, e.g.*, Andrews, "My Body My Property," 35; Hardiman, "Toward the Right of Commerciality," 238.

24. This was also the argument accepted in Miles, Inc. v. Scripps Clinic and Research Found., 810 F.Supp. at 1097–98.

25. See 35 U.S.C. (1988).

26. "Thus the patent system is one in which uniform federal standards are carefully used to promote invention while at the same time preserving free competition." Sears, Roebuck & Co. v. Stiffel Co., 376 U.S. 225, 230–31 (1964). See also ibid, 229–30.

27. 221 P.2d 73 (Cal. 1950).

28. 844 F.2d 988 (2nd Cir. 1988).

29. The majority held, in fact, that the individual components of Stanley's idea were not novel; only the combination was creative. Stanley v. Columbia Broadcasting System, Inc., 221 P.2d at 79.

30. Ibid., 79, 80.

31. If the majority had any of these ways of valuing Stanley's program idea in mind, it could not have made the statement that: "There is evidence to show that plaintiff's idea was of *no value whatsoever* to him after its use by the defendant." Ibid., 81 (emphasis added).

32. Stanley v. Columbia Broadcasting System, Inc., 221 P.2d at 84 (Traynor, J., dissenting).

33. Justice Traynor linked the free flow of abstract ideas with freedom:

[The law] does something more to stimulate creative activity: it assures all men [and women] free utilization of abstract ideas in the process of crystallizing them in fresh forms. For creativeness thrives on freedom;

men [and women] find new implications in old ideas when they range with open minds through open fields. They would indeed be stifled in their efforts to create forms worth protecting, if in the common through which they ranged they were diverted from their course by one enclosure after another.

Ibid.

34. Ibid., 85. Justice Traynor found support for his conclusions in an earlier case:

If an author, by originating a new arrangement and form of expression of certain ideas or conception, could withdraw these ideas or conceptions from the stock of materials to be used by other authors, each copyright would narrow the field of thought open for development and exploitation, and science, poetry, narrative, and dramatic fiction and other branches of literature would be hindered by copyright, instead of being promoted.

Ibid. (quoting Eichel v. Marein, 241 F. 404, 408–09 [U.S.D.C.N.Y. 1913]).
35. Ibid., 88–90.
36. To be more precise, Justice Traynor held that most of Stanley's program idea was valuable because it copied existing programming. The only portion of the idea that could plausibly be considered novel, Justice Traynor continued, was not copied by CBS. Ibid., 94. Given that Stanley had no property right to the "hackneyed" portions of his idea, CBS was free to copy them. Ibid.
37. Justice Traynor specifically eschewed the contemplation of aesthetic value: "It is not for the courts to consider the quality of an idea or to pass judgment on the public's taste; the problem before it is not one of aesthetics but of property rights." Ibid., 90.
38. 844 F.2d 988 (2nd Cir. 1988).
39. Ibid., 993–95. The majority recognized, however, that no idea is completely original; every idea is based on what has happened before: "We recognize of course that even novel and original ideas to a greater or lesser extent combine elements that are themselves not novel. Originality does not exist in a vacuum." Ibid., 993.
40. Ibid., 989, 992–93. The majority stated its conclusion as to the lack of novelty as follows:

We certainly do not dispute the fact that the portrayal of a nonstereotypical black family on television was indeed a breakthrough. Nevertheless, that breakthrough represents the achievement of what many black Americans, including Bill Cosby and plaintiff himself, have recognized for many years—namely, the need for a more positive, fair and realistic portrayal of blacks on television.

Ibid., 992.

41. Murray v. National Broadcasting Co., 844 F.2d at 997 (Pratt, J., dissenting.)

42. 248 U.S. 215 (1918).

43. Counsel for AP argued, for example, that AP "at large cost has established and operates an organization of labor and capital covering the whole world, and the product of this effort and expense is its property, because it made it." Int'l News Serv. v. Assoc. Press, 248 U.S. at 221–22.

44. INS employed strictly economic arguments in countering AP's claim to a property right in news. INS argued, essentially, that AP had given up any property right it may have had in the news when it permitted its east coast member papers to publish the news. INS did not contend that values, other than market values, were at stake in the case. Further, in stating that "[a] property right is not dependent upon its commercial value," ibid., 219–20, counsel for INS was not denying that a good must have a commercial value before it ought to be recognized as property; counsel was simply asserting that commercial value is not a sufficient condition to the recognition of a property right, since an individual can renounce a right to a good despite the good being commercially valuable.

45. The majority clearly recognized that INS and AP valued news as a commodity:

> For, to both of [INS and AP] alike, news matter, however little suscepti-
> ble of ownership or dominion in the absolute sense, is stock in trade,
> to be gathered at the cost of enterprise, organization, skill, labor, and
> money, and to be distributed and sold to those who will pay money
> for it, as for any other merchandise.

Ibid., 236.

46. The majority focused on the business aspect of collecting and distributing news:

> What we are concerned with is the business of making [news] known
> to the world, in which both parties to the present suit are engaged.
> That business consists in maintaining a prompt, sure, steady, and reli-
> able service designed to place the daily events of the world at the
> breakfast table of the millions at a price that, while of trifling moment
> to each reader, is sufficient in the aggregate to afford compensation for
> the cost of gathering and distributing it, with the added profit so neces-
> sary as an incentive to effective action in the commercial world.

Ibid., 235.

47. Ibid., 230–31, 238, 239.

48. Although the majority did not define in which ways news was valuable to the public, other than to say that the provision of news was "extremely useful," ibid., presumably readers valued news to satisfy their curiosity, to plan their futures and, given that the news in question dealt with the war, to keep track of the fate of their country and loved ones fighting in the war.

49. The majority carefully separated the claims of news agencies as against each other from claims of a news service against the public:

> Regarding the news, therefore, as but the material out of which both parties are seeking to make profits at the same time and in the same field, we hardly can fail to recognize that for this purpose, and as between them, it must be regarded as *quasi* property, irrespective of the rights of either as against the public.

Ibid., 236.

50. I leave out Justice Holmes's discussion of property rights in news. His discussion is short and the bases for his decision are unclear. While stating that property is a legal creation, Justice Holmes did not suggest how a court ought to decide whether to create it. His analysis that news is not property provides little insight into why it is not so and what requirement it would have to meet in order to be considered property:

> When an uncopyrighted combination of words is published there is no general right to forbid other people repeating them—in other words there is no property in the combination or in the thoughts or facts that the words express. Property, a creation of law, does not arise from value, although exchangeable—a matter of fact. Many exchangeable values may be destroyed intentionally without compensation. Property depends upon exclusion by law from interference, and a person is not excluded from using any combination of words merely because someone has used it before, even if it took labor and genius to make it.

Int'l News Serv. v. Assoc. Press, 248 U.S. at 246. Justice Holmes may have been concerned with the effect that a property right would likely have on the dissemination of ideas or on the fact that the entire field of property rights in words was occupied by legislation dealing with copyrights. His opinion does not, however, illuminate which, if either, of these concerns underlay his opposition to the recognition of property rights in news.

51. Justice Brandeis spoke of public interests rather than noneconomic interests, as I do. The meaning of the two phrases is, I submit, the same. Although the term "public interests" could be all-encompassing, Justice Brandeis contrasted it with "private interests." Since the term "private interests," in ordinary parlance, generally refers to interests that fall within a good's market price, Justice Brandeis was attempting to exclude market interests from his definition of "public interests." See ibid., 250, 262–63.

52. Int'l News Serv. v. Assoc. Press, 248 U.S. at 250, 262–63 (Brandeis, J., dissenting).

53. Justice Brandeis's concern over judicial competency ultimately grounded his decision to dissent from the grant of property, or quasiproperty, rights to AP:

> Courts are ill-equipped to make the investigations which should precede a determination of the limitations which should be set upon any property right in news or of the circumstances under which news gathered by a private agency should be deemed affected with a public interest. Courts would be powerless to prescribe the detailed regulations essential to full enjoyment of the rights conferred or to introduce the machinery required for enforcement of such regulations. Considerations such as these should lead us to decline to establish a new rule of law in the effort to redress a newly-disclosed wrong, although the propriety of some remedy appears to be clear.

Ibid., 267. The approach adopted by Justice Brandeis, that the courts ought to refrain from granting property rights where more than economic interests are at stake, is similar to that of Justice Arabian in Moore v. Regents of the Univ. of Cal., 51 Cal 3d 120 (1990). In the latter case, Justice Arabian held, essentially, that property law could only deal with economic interests; where a good is valuable in ways beyond its market price, the courts ought to refrain from acting.

54. This argument is similar to that made by the majority in Stanley v. Columbia Broadcasting System, 221 P.2d 73, 79 (Cal. 1950) that those who have exercised skill, discretion, and creative effort ought to be rewarded with property rights. Other cases will be canvassed in later chapters. See discussion in chapters 4–6.

55. The majority constructed its argument in the following language:

> In doing this [INS], by its very act, admits that it is taking material that has been acquired by complainant as the result of organization and the expenditure of labor, skill, and money, and which is saleable by [AP] for money, and that [INS] in appropriating it and selling it as its own is endeavoring to reap where it has not sown, and by disposing of it to newspapers that are competitors of [AP]'s members is appropriating to itself the harvest of those who have sown. Stripped of all disguises, the process amounts to an unauthorized interference with the normal operation of complainant's legitimate business precisely at the point where the profit is to be reaped, in order to divert a material portion of the profit from those who have earned it to those who have not; with special advantage to [INS] in the competition because of the fact that it is not burdened with any part of the expense of gathering news.

Int'l News Serv. v. Assoc. Press, 248 U.S. at 239–40.

56. Douglas G. Baird, "Common Law Intellectual Property and the Legacy of International News Service v. Associated Press," *University of Chicago Law Review* 50 (1983): 413; Weinrib, "Information and Property," 124.

57. This is not to say, of course, that the use made of the news by one individual may not reduce the market value of the news for another. But the fact that one individual's activity may reduce the price of news for another does not preclude the ability of that other to use the news as he or she wants: for example, by sharing it with family or by savoring it.

58. Baird, "Common Law Intellectual Property," 413.

59. The point can be made more general. In a market economy, the person who imitates the business of an individual who painstakingly planned the nature and location of her or his business does no injustice even if the competitor is able to siphon off much of the pioneer's profit. Ibid., 414; Weinrib, "Information and Property," 124.

60. "Whatsoever then he removes out of the state that nature hath provided, and left it in, he hath mixed his *labour* with, and joined to it something that is his own, and thereby makes it his *property*." John Locke, *Second Treatise of Government*, ed. C.B. Macpherson (Indianapolis: Hackett Publishers Co., 1980), p. 19 (¶27).

61. For criticism of Locke's view, see generally Jeremy Waldron, *The Right of Private Property* (Oxford: Clarendon Press, 1988).

62. See Weinrib, "Information and Property," 124.

63. See Int'l News Serv. v. Assoc. Press, 248 U.S. at 235, 238.

64. The market value of news, the majority held, is dependent on the novelty, freshness, reliability, and thoroughness of the news. Ibid., 238. See also ibid., 241.

65. This is not to say that the majority completely failed to acknowledge the existence of such values. The majority did state, after all, that news was socially important. Ibid., 235.

66. Remember that the majority, in determining whether all parties valued news in strictly economic terms, had cleaved off the dispute between the two news agencies from potential disputes between members of the public and one of these agencies. Here, in contrast, the majority put aside the public's interest in the existing dispute between the two news agencies. Taken together, these two positions put out of play any argument based on a third party interest in news itself or in the way in which news services collect and distribute news.

67. "But the fact that a product of the mind has cost its producer money and labor, and has a value for which others are willing to pay, is not sufficient to ensure to it this legal attribute of property." Int'l News Serv. v. Assoc. Press, 248 U.S. at 250 (Brandeis, J., dissenting). In a similar vein, Justice Brandeis wrote that:

> He who follows the pioneer into a new market, or who engages in the manufacture of an article newly introduced by another, seeks profits due largely to the labor and expense of the first adventurer; but the law sanctions, indeed encourages, the pursuit. He who makes a city

known through his product, must submit to sharing the resultant trade with others who, perhaps for that reason, locate there later.

Ibid., 259. See also ibid, 263.

68. Justice Brandeis emphasized the injustice that a monopoly in news would have:

The closing to the International News Service of these channels for foreign news (if they are closed) was due not to unwillingness on its part to pay the cost of collecting the news, but to the prohibitions imposed by foreign governments upon its securing news from their respective countries and from using cable or telegraph lines running therefrom. For aught that appears, this prohibition may have been wholly undeserved; and at all events the 400 papers and their readers may be assumed to have been innocent. For aught that appears, the International News Service may have sought then to secure temporarily by arrangement with the Associated Press the latter's foreign news service. For aught that appears all of the 400 subscribers of the International News Service would gladly have then become members of the Associated Press, if they could have secured election thereto. It is possible, also, that a large part of the readers of these papers were so situated that they could not secure prompt access to papers served by the Associated Press.

Ibid., 263–64.

69. 221 P.2d 73 (Cal. 1950).

70. 844 F.2d 988 (2nd Cir. 1988).

CHAPTER 4 NOTES

1. Mary Shelley, *Frankenstein: or the Modern Prometheus*, ed. Marilyn Butler (Oxford: Oxford University Press, 1994), pp. 38–39.

2. Following Mary Shelley's book of 1818, the Frankenstein story has spawned more than 26 films, the first in 1910, and 2 television movies. Susan King, "Karloff, Chaney, Lugosi and All the Rest," *Los Angeles Times*, 13 June 1993, p. 5(TV Times).

3. This fear is illustrated by those characters, such as Dr. Frankenstein's fiancee and friends, who viewed the creation of a new being as immoral.

4. The change in the monster's behavior, from innocent to evildoer, is brought about by the abuse he suffered at the hands of society.

5. There were two new versions, one for television and one on film, made in 1993. See Patricia Brennan, "Randy Quaid as Frankenstein's Monster," *Washington Post*, 13 June 1993, p. 5(Y); Michael Blowen, "Five-Minute Career Move," *Boston Globe*, 15 June 1993, p. 54(Living). In 1994, another big-budget motion picture was released. See Janet Maslin, "Frankenstein: A Brain on Ice, A Dead Toad and Voila!," *New York Times*, 4 November 1994, p. 1(C).

6. Bonito Boats, Inc. v. Thunder Craft Boats, Inc., 489 U.S. 141, 151 (1989).

7. Kewanee Oil Co. v. Bicron Co., 416 U.S. 470, 480 (1974).

8. 35 U.S.C. §§ 101–03 (1988).

9. See Brenner v. Manson, 383 U.S. 519, 534 (1965). But cf. Eisenberg, "Genes, Patents, and Product Development," 905.

10. Adler, "Genome Research," 911.

11. Kiley, "Patents on Random Complementary DNA Fragments?," 916; Eisenberg, "Genes, Patents, and Product Development," 905.

12. Bonito Boats, Inc. v. Thunder Craft Boats, Inc., 489 U.S. 141, 150.

13. See Brenner v. Manson, 383 U.S. at 518–19, 536.

14. See ibid., 534–35; Bonito Boats, Inc. v. Thunder Craft Boats, Inc., 489 U.S. at 146, 150–51.

15. This is much the same reason that underlies the courts' assumption that a contested invention must be useful. See discussion p. 66.

16. Phenomena of nature are those goods the qualities of which "are the work of nature." Funk Bros. Seed Co. v. Kalo Co., 333 U.S. 127, 130 (1947).

17. 248 U.S. 215 (1918).

18. See discussion pp. 56–59.

19. See, e.g., Gottschalk v. Benson, 409 U.S. 63, 67 (1972). See discussion pp. 71–74.

20. See discussion p. 44.

21. Remember that in Stanley v. Columbia Broadcasting Sys., Inc., 221 P.2d 73 (Cal. 1950) and Murray v. Nat'l Broadcasting Co., 844 F.2d 988 (2nd Cir. 1988) the majorities and dissents all agreed that only a particular concrete form of a program idea was entitled to copyright protection, not the entire idea. See also discussion pp. 49–53.

22. 409 U.S. 63 (1972).

23. The formula set out how to calculate the pure binary equivalent of a sequence of binary numbers, each of which represents one digit of a decimal number. For example, the two binary numbers 0101 (5 in decimal) and 0011 (3 in decimal) are converted into the pure binary number 110101 (53 in decimal).

24. Gottschalk v. Benson, 409 U.S. at 68, 70, 72.

25. Ibid., 67.

26. The Court, in discussing an earlier decision dealing with Samuel Morse's claim to a patent in all electromagnetic forms of communication at a distance, pointed to the dangers of granting patent rights in phenomena of nature:

> For aught that we now know, some future inventor, in the onward march of science, may discover a mode of writing or printing at a distance by means of the electric or galvanic current, without using any part of the process or combination set forth in the plaintiff's specification. His invention may be less complicated—less liable to get out of order—

less expensive in construction, and in its operation. But yet, if it is covered by this patent, the inventor could not use it, nor the public have the benefit of it, without the permission of this patentee.

Gottschalk v. Benson, 409 U.S. at 68 (quoting O'Reilly v. Morse, 15 How. 62, 113 (U.S.S.C. 1853)).

27. This proposition was asserted forcefully by the Court in a case that will be discussed later:

The qualities of these bacteria, like the heat of the sun, electricity, or the qualities of metals, are part of the storehouse of knowledge of all men. They are manifestations of laws of nature, free to all men and reserved exclusively to none. He who discovers a hitherto unknown phenomenon of nature has no claim to a monopoly of it which the law recognizes.

Funk Bros. Seed Co. v. Kalo Co., 333 U.S. 127, 130 (1947).

28. See Locke, *Second Treatise of Government*, 19 (¶27); see also Waldron, *The Right of Private Property*, 140–41.

29. 248 U.S. 215 (1918).

30. See discussion pp. 56–59.

31. Gottschalk v. Benson, 409 U.S. at 72–73.

32. 437 U.S. 584 (1978).

33. See ibid., 589, 591–92, 594.

34. See ibid., 590.

35. The Court stated:

The notion that post-solution activity, no matter how conventional or obvious in itself, can transform an unpatentable principle into a patentable process exalts form over substance. A competent draftsman could attach some form of post-solution activity to almost any mathematical formula; the Pythagorean theorem would have been patentable, or partially patentable, because a patent application contained a final step indicating that the formula, when solved, could be usefully applied to existing surveying techniques.

Parker v. Flook, 437 U.S. at 590.

36. See ibid., 594.

37. Ibid., 595.

38. See, e.g., ibid., 593.

39. 450 U.S. 175 (1981).

40. The dissent in *Diehr* held that this was the central issue in the case. Diamond v. Diehr, 450 U.S. at 207 (Stevens, J., dissenting).

41. Diamond v. Diehr, 450 U.S. at 181.

42. Parker v. Flook, 437 U.S. at 594–95.

43. The dissent wrote:

> [W]hat Diehr and Lutton claim to have discovered is a method of using a digital computer to determine the amount of time that a rubber molding press should remain closed during the synthetic rubber-curing process. There is no suggestion that there is anything novel in the instrumentation of the mold, in actuating a timer when the press is closed, or in automatically opening the press when the computer time expires.

Diamond v. Diehr, 450 U.S. at 208 (Stevens, J., dissenting). See also ibid, 209.

44. Diamond v. Diehr, 450 U.S. at 184, 187, 192.

45. One must remember that both *Benson* and *Flook* had already moved considerably from the moral core of the phenomena of nature argument.

46. It is worth noting that, in arguing against the grant of Diehr's claims, the dissent in *Diehr* employed the institutional competency argument introduced in both *Benson* and *Flook*. As in those cases, the dissent held that difficult policy issues surrounded the question of whether computer programs and algorithms ought to be patentable. These issues, the dissent stated, were outside the competency of the courts to address. Diamond v. Diehr, 450 U.S. at 216–17 (Stevens, J., dissenting). It was unclear, the dissent continued, what economic effect the award of patent rights in programs and algorithms would have. Ibid., 217–18. In addition, the dissent warned, serious administrative problems were likely to arise within the Patent and Trademark Office should it be flooded with patent applications covering algorithms and programs. Ibid., 218.

47. 333 U.S. 118 (1947).

48. 447 U.S. 303 (1980).

49. Funk Bros. Seed Co. v. Kalo Co., 333 U.S. at 130–32.

50. The Court was adamant on this point:

> But once nature's secret of the non-inhibitive quality of certain strains of the species of *Rhizobium* was discovered, the state of the art made the production of a mixed inoculant a simple step. Even though it may have been the product of skill, it certainly was not the product of invention. There is no way in which we could call it such unless we borrowed invention from the discovery of the natural principle itself. That is to say, there is no invention here unless the discovery that certain strains of the several species of these bacteria are non-inhibitive and may thus be safely mixed is invention.

Ibid., 132.

51. Eisenberg, "Genes, Patents, and Product Development," 904.

52. 447 U.S. 303 (1980).

53. Ibid., 309 (quoting S. Rep. No. 1979, 82d Cong., 2d Sess. 5 (1952) and H.R. Rep. No. 1923, 82d Cong., 2d Sess. 6 (1952)).

54. Ibid., 307 (quoting Kewanee Oil Co. v. Bicron Co., 416 U.S. 470, 480 [1974]).

55. See ibid., 309–13.

56. Ibid., 316–17. See generally Sharon Kingman, "Safety Concerns Halt U.K. Study," *Science* 263 (1994): 748; Eliot Marshall, "One Less Hoop for Gene Therapy," *Science* 265 (1994): 599.

57. Diamond v. Chakrabarty, 447 U.S. at 317.

58. Ibid. This statement ignores the hope of those opposed to genetic research to slow down its pace. See ibid., 316.

59. Ibid., 315, 317–18.

60. For example, one may well wonder about the consistency of stating that patent rights are immaterial to the progress of science when the Court's rationale for awarding such rights is that they are needed to encourage scientific development.

61. Weinrib, "Information and Property," 121; see also discussion p. 44.

62. Diamond v. Chakrabarty, 447 U.S. at 317.

63. This is, in some measure, the argument made by the dissent. Diamond v. Chakrabarty, 447 U.S. at 322 (Brennan, J., dissenting).

64. Diamond v. Chakrabarty, 447 U.S. at 317.

CHAPTER 5 NOTES

1. "'I'll Swap You 2 'Hound Dogs' for . . .': Elvis Trading Cards Fuel His Fans' 'Burning Love'," *New York Times*, 28 August 1992, p. 3(D).

2. Factors Etc., Inc. v. Pro Arts, Inc., 579 F.2d 215, 216 (2d Cir., 1978).

3. For example, consider the work of Audrey Hepburn on behalf of U.N.I.C.E.F. and Elizabeth Taylor's efforts to raise money to combat AIDS.

4. In addition to Elvis, many celebrities, including Elizabeth Taylor, Johnny Carson, and Lee Iacocca have used their fame to sell commercial products.

5. Price v. Hal Roach Studios, Inc., 400 F.Supp. 836, 843–44 (S.D.N.Y. 1975).

6. Tennessee *ex rel.* Elvis Presley Int'l Memorial Found. v. Crowell, 733 S.W.2d 89, 94 (Tenn. Ct. App. 1987).

7. Waits v. Frito-Lay, Inc., 978 F.2d 1093, 1098 (9th Cir. 1992).

8. Martin Luther King, Jr., Ctr. for Social Change, Inc. v. American Heritage Prods., Inc., 694 F.2d 674, 680 (11th Cir. 1983).

9. Price v. Hal Roach Studios, Inc., 400 F.Supp. at 844.

10. See Martin Luther King, Jr., Ctr. for Social Change v. American Heritage Prods., Inc., 694 F.2d at 680; Waits v. Frito-Lay, Inc., 978 F.2d 1093, 1102–6.

11. See Carson v. Here's Johnny Portable Toilets, Inc., 698 F.2d 831, 834 (6th Cir. 1983).

12. Price v. Hal Roach Studios, Inc., 400 F.Supp. at 844–46; Factors Etc., Inc. v. Pro Arts, Inc., 579 F.2d 215, 220–21 (2d Cir. 1978); Tennessee *ex rel.* Elvis Presley Int'l Memorial Found. v. Crowell, 733 S.W. 2d at 97–99;

Martin Luther King., Jr., Ctr. for Social Change v. American Heritage Prods. Inc., at 680–83; see also Lugosi v. Universal Pictures, 603 P.2d 425, 429–30 (Cal. 1979). Contra Memphis Dev. Found. v. Factors Etc., Inc., 616 F.2d 956 (6th Cir. 1980).

13. This is assuming, of course, that the celebrity had not sold or transferred this right to another during his or her life.

14. Price v. Hal Roach Studios, Inc., 400 F.Supp. at 844. But cf. Martin Luther King, Jr., Ctr. for Social Change, Inc. v. American Heritage Prods., 694 F.2d at 677.

15. Waits v. Frito-Lay, Inc., 978 F.2d 1093, 1098 (9th Cir. 1992); see also Zacchini v. Scripps-Howard Broadcasting Co., 433 US. 562, 573 (1976). But cf. Lugosi v. Universal Pictures, 603 P.2d at 428.

16. George M. Armstrong, Jr., "The Reification of Celebrity: Persona as Property," *Louisiana Law Review* 51 (1991): 443.

17. Cf. Memphis Dev. Found. v. Factors Etc., Inc., 616 F.2d 956, 958 (6th Cir. 1980).

18. Carson v. Here's Johnny Portable Toilets, Inc., 698 F.2d 831, 835 (6th Cir. 1983).

19. See Zacchini v. Scripps-Howard Broadcasting Co., 433 U.S. at 573. While one only values the commercial aspects of one's persona in terms of market price, the decision to treat one's persona as a commodity raises other values:

> The very decision to exploit name and likeness is a personal one. It is not at all unlikely that Lugosi and others in his position did not during their respective lifetimes exercise their undoubted right to capitalize upon their personalities, and transfer the value thereof into some commercial venture, for reasons of taste or judgment or because the enterprise to be organized might be too demanding or simply because they did not want to be bothered.

Lugosi v. Universal Pictures, 603 P.2d at 430.

20. 51 Cal. 3d 120 (1990). See chapter 2.

21. 248 U.S. 215 (1918). See chapter 3.

22. 447 U.S. 303 (1980). See discussion p. 81.

23. Zacchini v. Scripps-Howard Broadcasting Co., 433 U.S. at 567. See also Carson v. Here's Johnny Portable Toilets, Inc., 698 F.2d at 837; Martin Luther King, Jr., Ctr. for Social Change v. American Heritage Prods., 694 F.2d at 682.

24. Zacchini v. Scripps-Howard Broadcasting Co., 433 U.S. at 573. See also Tennessee *ex rel.* Elvis Presley Int'l Memorial Found. v. Crowell, 733 S.W.2d at 98.

25. The dissent in Lugosi v. Universal Pictures, 603 P.2d 425, 441–42 (Cal. 1979) (Bird, C.J., dissenting) came closest to stating why public personae are valuable:

> While the immediate beneficiaries are those who establish professions or identities which are commercially valuable, the products of their

enterprise are often beneficial to society generally. Their performances, inventions and endeavors enrich our society, while their participation in commercial enterprises may communicate valuable information to consumers.

Even this statement, however, fails to inform us in which ways performances are valuable.

Recall that this same problem arose with respect to the received learning that the label "property" represents the legal conclusion that a good is, in some way, valuable. See discussion p. 44. Just as the received learning failed to define in which way a good must be valuable in order to be considered property, the courts' holding that the creation of public personae is beneficial to society fails to explain in which ways such personae are beneficial.

26. Consider the following statement: "Unquestionably, a celebrity's right of publicity has value. It can be possessed and used. It can be assigned, and it can be the subject of contract." Tennessee *ex rel.* Elvis Presley Int'l Memorial Found. v. Crowell, 733 S.W.2d at 97. This analysis of why personae are valuable points to the instrumental stance taken by the court with respect to such personae. That is, the court valued personae simply as instruments to be bought and sold; it ignored the intrinsic value of personae, such as their importance to self-esteem, self-development, and human dignity.

27. See ibid.; Zacchini v. Scripps-Howard Broadcasting Co., 433 U.S. at 572; Memphis Dev. Found. v. Factors Etc., Inc., 616 F.2d at 958; Carson v. Here's Johnny Portable Toilets, 698 F.2d at 835.

28. Martin Luther King, Jr., Ctr. for Social Change v. American Heritage Prods., 694 F.2d at 683.

29. Lugosi v. Universal Pictures, 603 P.2d 425, 439 n.11 (Cal. 1979) (Bird, C.J., dissenting).

30. In *King*, the court only noted this effect toward the end of its opinion. Even then, the court resorted to a footnote to explain that, instead of the economic argument it presented, it could have sustained the entire right of publicity on the basis of such noneconomic values. Martin Luther King, Jr., Ctr. for Social Change v. American Heritage Prods., 694 F.2d at 683 n.6. In *Lugosi*, the dissent recognized that the right of publicity furthers noneconomic values. As the court in *King*, however, the dissent did so only in a footnote and only after having supported the right of publicity solely on economic grounds. Lugosi v. Universal Pictures, 603 P.2d at 439 n.11.

31. Zacchini v. Scripps-Howard Broadcasting Co., 433 U.S. at 573.

32. 248 U.S. 215 (1918).

33. Lugosi v. Universal Pictures, 603 P.2d at 438 (Bird, C.J., dissenting); Tennessee *ex rel.* Elvis Presley Int'l Memorial Found. v. Crowell, 733 S.W.2d at 98.

34. See discussion pp. 56–59.

35. Consider, for example, the following statement:

Of course, Ohio's decision to protect petitioner's right of publicity here rests on more than a desire to compensate the performer for the time and effort invested in his act; the protection provides the economic incentive for him to make the investment required to produce a performance of interest to the public.

Zacchini v. Scripps-Howard Broadcasting Co., 433 U.S. at 576.
   36. Ibid.
   37. U.S. Const. amend. I.
   38. Zacchini v. Scripps-Howard Broadcasting Co., 433 U.S. at 578.
   39. See ibid., 573.
   40. Ibid., 575.
   41. Ibid., 575 n.12.
   42. See Armstrong, "The Reification of Celebrity," 443.
   43. See Price v. Hal Roach Studios, Inc., 400 F.Supp. 836, 844 (S.D.N.Y. 1975).
   44. Ibid. The right of publicity thus contrasts with the right of privacy. The latter right, based solely on the right-holder's feelings, properly dies with the right-holder. Ibid.
   45. See Factors Etc., Inc. v. Pro Art, Inc., 579 F.2d 215 (2nd Cir. 1978).
   46. Tennessee *ex rel.* Elvis Presley Int'l Memorial Found. v. Crowell, 733 S.W.2d 89, 98 (Tenn. Ct. App. 1987).
   47. 616 F.2d 956 (6th Cir. 1980).
   48. Ibid., 957–58.
   49. Specifically, the court stated:

Heretofore, the law has always thought that leaving a good name to one's children is sufficient reward in itself for the individual, whether famous or not. Commercialization of this virtue after death in the hands of heirs is contrary to our legal tradition and somehow seems contrary to the moral presuppositions of our culture.

Ibid., 959.
   50. Ibid, 959–60. The court probably misunderstood Factors's argument. Factors's argument was that the present value of one's right of publicity is increased if the right survives one's death. Therefore, one can sell this right, during one's life, for more money than one would receive if the right terminated at one's death. Thus, the incentive provided by the survivability of the right of publicity accrues to the creator of the persona, not to the creator's heirs. The question the court ought to have asked was whether this incentive was sufficient to motivate more creation.
   51. 579 F.2d 215 (2d Cir.1978), effectively overturned by Factors Etc., Inc. v. Pro Arts, Inc. 652 F.2d 278 (2d Cir. 1981) on a different issue.
   52. Ibid., 221.
   53. 733 S.W.2d 89 (Tenn. Ct. App. 1987).
   54. Remember that *Memphis Development* was decided by the United States Court of Appeals for the Sixth Circuit applying Tennessee law. *Crowell*, in contrast, was actually decided by a Tennessee court. Thus, the decision in *Crowell* effectively overruled the holding in *Memphis Development*.
   55. 733 S.W.2d at 97.

56. The court actually put forward six arguments in favor of its position. The first three arguments—that since the right of publicity was a personal property right before death, it should remain a property right after death, that one ought not reap where one has not sown, and that descendibility vindicates the celebrity's expectation that she or he is creating a valuable capital asset—amount to the broad argument that individuals must be given a financial incentive in order to create. The last three arguments—that recognizing the right of publicity to be descendible protects the interests of those who have contracted for this right, that a monopoly over the use of a celebrity's persona protects the public against deception, and that descendibility protects against unfair competition—amount to the argument that individuals will not invest in another's persona unless the market value of that persona is stable. If the right to use that persona terminates at the celebrity's death, then that market value will be too uncertain to attract investment.

57. Consider the following statement:

> While a celebrity's expectation that his heirs will benefit from his right of publicity might not, by itself, provide a basis to recognize that the right of publicity is descendible, it does recognize the effort and financial commitment celebrities make in their careers. This investment deserves no less recognition and protection than investments celebrities might make in the stock market or in other tangible assets.

Ibid., 98.

58. Ibid., 98.

59. 603 P.2d 425, 428, 430–31 (Cal. 1979).

60. The following passage illustrates the majority's trust in market forces to encourage the creation of personae:

> Thus, under present law, upon Lugosi's death, anyone, related or unrelated to Lugosi, with the imagination, the enterprise, the energy and the cash could, in his or her own name or in a fictitious name, or a trade name coupled with that of Lugosi, have impressed a name so selected with a secondary meaning and realized a profit or loss by so doing depending upon the value of the idea, its acceptance by the public and the management of the enterprise undertaken.

Ibid., 430.

61. The grant of a property right to celebrities who exploit their personae provides this kind of incentive since the property right survives the celebrity:

> Assuming arguendo that Lugosi, in his lifetime, based upon publicity he received and/or because of the nature of his talent in exploiting his name and likeness in association with the Dracula character, had established a business under the name of Lugosi Horror Pictures and sold licenses to have "Lugosi as Dracula" imprinted on shirts, and in so doing built a large public acceptance and/or good will for such business,

product or service, there is little doubt that Lugosi would have created during his lifetime a business or property wholly apart from the rights he had granted Universal to exploit his name and likeness in the characterization of the lead role of Count Dracula in the picture, *Dracula*.

Ibid., 429.

62. Lugosi v. Universal Pictures, 603 P.2d 425, 446–47 (Cal. 1979) (Bird, C.J., dissenting).

63. 694 F.2d 674 (11th Cir. 1983).

64. 296 S.E.2d 697 (Ga. 1982) reproduced in the Eleventh Circuit's reasons. I will be referring throughout to the version the Supreme Court of Georgia's reasons reproduced as an exhibit to the Eleventh Circuit's opinion.

65. The court's desire to encourage the production of personae is illustrated in the following:

Recognition of the right of publicity rewards and thereby encourages effort and creativity. If the right of publicity dies with the celebrity, the economic value of the right of publicity during life would be diminished because the celebrity's untimely death would seriously impair, if not destroy, the value of the right of continued commercial use.

694 F.2d at 682.

66. See, e.g., ibid., 680, 681–82, 683.

67. Ibid., 683 n.6.

68. This is particularly true in the case of King, who devoted himself to the public good:

Perhaps this case more than others brings the point into focus. A well known minister may avoid exploiting his prominence during life because to do otherwise would impair his ministry. . . In our view, a person who avoids exploitation during life is entitled to have his image protected against exploitation after death just as much if not more than a person who exploited his image during life.

Ibid., 683.

69. Waits v. Frito-Lay, Inc., 978 F.2d 1093 (9th Cir. 1992).

70. Carson v. Here's Johnny Portable Toilets, Inc., 698 F.2d 831 (6th Cir. 1983).

71. 698 F.2d 831 (6th Cir. 1983).

72. Ibid., 835, 837.

73. Carson v. Here's Johnny Portable Toilets, Inc., 698 F.2d 831, 838–39 (6th Cir. 1983) (Kennedy, J., dissenting).

74. Ibid., 840. The dissent, in continuing this argument, stated that words and ideas ought to remain in public circulation unless a specific law requires otherwise. Ibid., 841. Words and ideas have generally been regarded, the dissent maintained, as being too abstract to qualify for property protection.

Their ownership closes off too great an area of endeavor from other creators. Cf. Sears, Roebuck & Co. v. Stiffel Co., 376 U.S. 225. See also chapter 3.

75. Carson v. Here's Johnny Portable Toilets, Inc. 698 F.2d at 840.

76. The dissent characterized this difficulty as the failure to provide adequate notice:

> As the right of privacy [sic] is expanded beyond protections of name, likeness and actual performances, which provide relatively objective notice to the public of the extent of an individual's rights, to more subjective attributes such as achievements and identifying characteristics, the public's ability to be on notice of a common law monopoly right, if one is even asserted by a given famous individual, is severely diminished.

Ibid.

77. 433 U.S. 502 (1977).

78. See, e.g., Hudnut v. American Bookseller's Ass'n, 475 U.S. 1001 (1986); Village of Skokie v. National Socialist Party of America, 366 N.E.2d 347 (Ill.App.Ct. 1977).

79. This placement of economic value well ahead of all others inhering in personae explains the difficulty that the *King* court encountered in drafting its reasons. In *King*, the court justified both the right of publicity and the descendibility of this right on the basis of the purely economic argument that individuals would not create personae without the economic incentive provided by the opportunity to commercially exploit those personae. In so doing, the *King* court simply followed the order of values implicit in property law: economic value on top, all others well below. Upon reaching the question of whether a celebrity must first exploit his or her persona before the right of publicity becomes descendible, however, the court reached the uncomfortable conclusion that some values were more important than economic value: specifically, society's respect for and memory of King. The court's discomfort did not induce it, however, to completely abandon its economic arguments. The court justified most of its holding on the basis of valuing King's persona as a market good; it deserted this basis only when it conflicted with the noneconomic values the court considered more important.

80. 978 F.2d 1093 (9th Cir. 1992).

81. As the court in *Waits* noted, this use of "Step Right Up" was ironic, given that the song parodied commercial hucksterism. Ibid., 1097.

82. Ibid., 1098–1100.

83. Recall the statement in Zacchini v. Scripps-Howard Broadcasting Co., 433 U.S. 562, 573 that the right of publicity focuses "on the right of the individual to reap the reward of his endeavors and [has] little to do with protecting feelings or reputation."

84. Waits v. Frito-Lay, Inc., 978 F.2d 1093, 1103).

85. See Motschenbacher v. R.J. Reynolds Tobacco Co., 498 P.2d 821, 824 n.11 (9th Cir. 1974); Lugosi v. Universal Pictures, 603 P.2d 425, 439 n.11 (Cal. 1979) (Bird, C.J., dissenting).

86. Waits v. Frito-Lay, Inc., 978 F.2d 1093.

87. See, e.g., Hirsch v. S.C. Johnson & Son, Inc., 280 N.W.2d 129 (Wis. 1979).

88. I am assuming, as the courts do, that selling records and concert tickets does not constitute the commercial exploitation of Waits's voice. Generally, only when a celebrity markets her or his persona as a good in itself—a poster, a belt buckle, or a signature—or a product to which the celebrity has attached his or her name is the celebrity considered to have commercially exploited his or her identity. Further, although Waits had an "interest" in the commercial aspects of his voice, it was the interest not to exploit it. Thus, for the purposes of this discussion, when I state that Waits had no commercial interest in his voice, I mean only that he did not value his voice because of its value in selling products; in fact, he shunned that value.

CHAPTER 6 NOTES

1. "Welcome and stay out," *The Economist*, 14 May 1994, 55.

2. See Stephen Kinzer, "Bonn Parliament Votes Sharp Curb on Asylum Seekers," *New York Times*, 27 May 1993, p. 1(A); Stephen Kinzer, "Rights Group Attack German Plan on Refugees," *New York Times*, 7 February 1993, p. 11(I); Stephen Kinzer, "Germany Agrees on Law to Curb Refugees and Seekers of Asylum," *New York Times*, 8 December 1992, p. 1(A); Craig Whitney, "Bonn Plans Curbs to Halt Refugees," *New York Times*, 14 October 1992, p. 1(A).

3. 447 U.S. 303 (1980).

4. 694 F.2d 674 (11th Cir. 1983).

5. See Waits v. Frito-Lay, Inc., 978 F.2d 1093 (9th Cir. 1992).

6. Compare Waits v. Frito-Lay, Inc., 978 F.2d 1093 with Stanley v. Columbia Broadcasting Sys., Inc., 221 P.2d 73 (Cal. 1950).

7. 538 F.2d 14 (2d Cir. 1976).

8. Ibid., 20, 21, 23, 24.

9. Ibid., 24–25. Monty Python's claim was one of moral right (*droit moral*), a right recognized in civil law countries.

10. Thus, the law considers the violation of artistic integrity as analogous to unfair competition: "This statute [Lanham Act, 15 U.S.C. § 1125(a)], the federal counterpart to state unfair competition laws, has been invoked to prevent misrepresentations that may injure plaintiff's business or personal reputation, even where no registered trademark is concerned." Ibid.

11. One need only think of the Impressionists as an illustration of this point.

12. Consider Andy Warhol's use of the artwork on the label of soup cans.

13. 248 U.S. 215 (1918).

14. 447 U.S. 303 (1980).

15. 433 U.S. 562 (1976).

16. 694 F.2d 674 (11th Cir. 1983).

17. 978 F.2d 1093 (9th Cir. 1992).

18. 631 F.2d 1264 (6th Cir. 1980).

19. As the trial judge observed:

Everything that has happened in the Mahoning Valley has been happening for many years because of steel. Schools have been built, roads have been built. Expansion that has taken place is because of steel. And to accommodate that industry, lives and destinies of the inhabitants of that community were based and planned on the basis of that institution: Steel.

Ibid., 1265.

20. Joseph W. Singer, "The Reliance Interest in Property," *Stanford Law Review* 40 (1988): 614–18.

21. Local 1330, United Steel Workers of America v. United States Steel Corp., 631 F.2d 1264, 1279–80 (6th Cir. 1980).

22. Ibid, 1266.

23. Ibid., 1280.

24. Like the district court, the court of appeals searched high and low for authority on which to base a property right for the community:

Our problem in dealing with plaintiff's fourth cause of action is one of authority. Neither in brief nor oral argument have plaintiffs pointed to any constitutional provision contained in either the Constitution of the United States or the Constitution of the State of Ohio, nor any law enacted by the United States Congress or the Legislature of Ohio, nor any case decided by the courts of either of these jurisdictions which would convey authority to this court to require the United States Steel Corporation to continue operations in Youngstown which its officers and Board of Directors had decided to discontinue on the basis of unprofitability.

Ibid.

25. Ibid., 1282.

26. Singer, "Reliance Interest in Property," 612 n.9.

27. Similarly, lenders may be wary of loaning money on the security of a plant the ownership of which is in doubt.

28. Weinrib, "Information and Property," 121; see also discussion p. 44.

29. Another community effort to block to shutdown of a plant, this time an automobile plant, similarly failed. Ypsilanti v. General Motors Corp., 506 N.W.2d 556 (Mich. Ct. App. 1993). The community did not seek a property right in the plant in that case.

30. 94 U.S. 113 (1877).

31. Local 1330, United Steel Workers v. United States Steel, 631 F.2d at 1282–83 (quoting Munn v. Illinois, 94 U.S. at 134).

32. Recall that the Court in Diamond v. Chakrabarty similarly relied on this judicial incompetency argument to avoid consideration of noneconomic values, in that case environmental safety and human health. Ibid., 317; see discussion p. 83.

33. Richard A. Posner, *The Economics of Justice* (Cambridge, Mass.: Harvard University Press, 1981), p. 71; Guido Calabresi and A. Douglas Melamed, "Property Rules, Liability Rules, and Inalienability: One View of the Cathedral," *Harvard Law Review* 85 (1972): 1100. Robin Hahnel and Michael Albert, *Quiet Revolution in Welfare Economics* (Princeton, N.J.: Princeton University Press, 1990), pp. 75–109 warns, however, that the traditional economic paradigm fails to take into account many externalities.

34. Calabresi and Melamed, "Property Rules," 1103, 1110; see also Guido Calabresi and Philip Bobbitt, *Tragic Choices* (New York: W.W. Norton & Co., 1978).

CHAPTER 7 NOTES

1. Eduardo Galeano, *The Book of Embraces*, trans. Cedric Belfrage (New York: W.W. Norton & Co., 1991), p. 140.

2. More precisely, Taylor invokes the landscape metaphor to discuss how we make decisions about our lives and the goods that affect our lives. Taylor, *Sources of the Self*, 28–29, 41–42.

3. Ibid., 26–28.

4. Ibid.

5. Although I do believe that at some level most apply to all cultures.

6. Michel Foucault, *Discipline & Punish: The Birth of the Prison*, trans. Alan Sheridan (New York: Vintage Books, 1979).

7. Nancy Fraser, "Foucault's Body-Language: A Post-Humanist Political Rhetoric?," *Salmagundi* 61 (1983): 64. See also Jana Sawicki, *Disciplining Foucault: Feminism, Power, and the Body* (New York: Routledge, 1991), p. 80.

8. See Ioan P. Culianu, "A Corpus for the Body," *Journal of Modern History* 63 (1991): 66.

9. David M. Levin and George F. Solomon, "The Discursive Formation of the Body in the History of Medicine," *Journal of Medicine and Philosophy* 15 (1990): 523. See Mark Kidel and Susan Rowe-Leete, "Mapping the Body," in *Fragments for a History of the Human Body*, ed. Michel Feher (New York: Zone, 1989), 3:465–66 for a pictorial illustration of the link between the body and the cosmos.

10. Jacques Le Goff, "Head or Heart? The Political Use of Body Metaphors in the Middle Ages, " in *Fragments for a History of the Human Body*, ed. Michel Feher (New York: Zone, 1989), 3:13; Randall McGowen, "The Body and Punishment in Eighteenth-Century England," *Journal of Modern History* 59 (1987): 654.

11. Women and other marginal groups were thought to be grotesque forms of this classic body. Laurie Finke, "Mystical Bodies and the Dialogics of Vision," *Philological Quarterly* 67 (1988): 444.

12. Le Goff, "Head or Heart?," 14.

13. Ibid., 16–17.

14. Levin and Solomon, "Discursive Formation of the Body," 519.

15. McGowen, "Body and Punishment," 67.

16. Pasi Falk, "Corporeality and Its Fates in History," *Acta Sociologica* 28, no. 2 (1985): 122.

17. Levin and Solomon, "Discursive Formation of the Body," 522–23.

18. Ibid., 524.

19. Scarry, *Body in Pain*, 109.

20. See the discussion of Lacan's mirror stage in Catherine Clément, *The Lives and Legends of Jacques Lacan*, trans. Arthur Goldhammer (New York: Columbia University Press, 1983), pp. 84–92.

21. Juliet Mitchell, *Psycho-Analysis and Feminism* (New York: Vintage Books, 1975), pp. 384–86.

22. Daniel C. Dennett, *Consciousness Explained* (Boston: Little, Brown and Co., 1991), p. 414.

23. Bruce M. Knauft, "Bodily Images in Melanesia: Cultural Substances and Natural Metaphors," in *Fragments for a History of the Human Body*, ed. Michel Feher (New York: Zone, 1989), pp. 223–25.

24. See Browning v. Norton-Children's Hospital, 504 S.W.2d 713 (Ky. 1974).

25. See Oliver Sacks, "The Man Who Fell Out of Bed," in *The Man Who Mistook his Wife for a Hat and Other Clinical Tales* (New York: Harper & Row, 1987), p. 55.

26. G. Hegel, *Philosophy of Right*, trans. T.M. Knox (New York: Oxford University Press, 1967), ¶47. (As the *Philosophy of Right* is divided into paragraphs, remarks to paragraphs and additions to paragraphs, "¶" followed by a number will refer to paragraph numbers and "¶" followed by a number and an "R" will refer to the remarks found beneath the paragraph indicated by the number.)

27. Ibid., ¶48R.

28. Foucault, *Discipline and Punish*, 25–30.

29. Genesis 2:24.

30. Genesis 24:9:

So the servant put his hand under the thigh of Abraham his master, and swore to him concerning this matter.

31. See, e.g., Pennzoil Co. v. Texaco Inc., 729 S.W.2d 768 (Tex. Ct. App. 1987).

32. This and the following two examples are discussed in Johan Huizinga, *The Waning of the Middle Ages* (New York: Doubleday & Co., 1954), p. 167.

33. John Kifner, "Amid Frenzy, Iranians Bury The Ayatollah," *New York Times*, 7 June 1989, p. 1(A).

34. Titmuss, *Gift Relationship*.

35. Thomas H. Murray, "Gifts of the Body and the Needs of Strangers," *Hastings Center Report*, April 1987, 30:36.

36. Genesis 1:27:

So God created man in his own image, in the image of God he created him; male and female he created them.

37. Genesis 9:4–5. See also Deuteronomy 12:16.
38. Genesis 4:10:

And the LORD said, "What have you done? The voice of your brother's blood is crying to me from the ground."

39. William I. Miller, "Choosing the Avenger: Some Aspects of the Bloodfeud in Medieval Iceland and England," *Law and History Review* 1 (1983): 182 n. 92.
40. Knauft, "Bodily Images in Melanesia," 235–36.
41. John 13:10.
42. Finke, "Mystical Bodies," 446–47.
43. Scarry, *Body in Pain*, 34.
44. Culianu, "Corpus for the Body," 65.
45. Finke, "Mystical Bodies," 447.
46. Culianu, "Corpus for the Body," 71.
47. Aristotle thought that the birth of a female child demonstrated some infirmity in the father. Giulia Sissa, "Subtle Bodies," in *Fragments for a History of the Human Body*, ed. Michel Feher (New York: Zone, 1989), p. 136.
48. Finke, "Mystical Bodies," 444.
49. Sissa, "Subtle Bodies," 139–40.
50. Luke 1:26–41.
51. Genesis 3:16.
52. Genesis 4:15.
53. See, e.g., Peter Steinfels, "AIDS Provokes Theological Second Thoughts," *New York Times*, 19 November 1989, p. 5(4); Edward Tivnan, "Homosexuals and the Churches," *New York Times*, 11 October 1987, p. 84(6).
54. Culianu, "Corpus for the Body," 78–79.
55. See Thomas Murray's discussion of the views of Joseph Fletcher and H. Tristam Engelhardt. Thomas H. Murray, "On the Human Body as Property: the Meaning of Embodiment, Markets, and the Meaning of Strangers," *Journal of Law Reform* 20 (1987): 1064–68.
56. McGowen, "The Body and Punishment," 651, 661, 664.
57. Albert Camus, *La Peste* (Paris: Gallimard, 1947).
58. Allen Thiher, "Teaching the Historical Context of *The Plague*," in *Approaches to Teaching Camus's The Plague*, ed. Steven G. Kellman (New York: Modern Language Association of America, 1985), pp. 95–97:

The Plague is perhaps most clearly referential in the way it documents the details of how daily life goes on in the face of an occupying army. The rationing of food, the hedonistic drinking, the reruns of films in the cinemas, the hoarding of scarce goods and the organizing of a black market, the closing of shops left abandoned by the "departed," the

imposing of curfews, the creation of "isolation camps" for mass intern-
ments, the inordinate demands made on one's physical stamina—these
and many other details offer exact parallels with life during the Occupation.

59. Alfons Labish, "The Social Construction of Health: From Early Modern Times to the Beginnings of the Industrialization," in *The Social Construction
of Illness: Illness and Medical Knowledge in Past and Present*, ed. Jens Lachmund
and Gunnar Stollberg (Stuttgart, Germ.: Franz Steiner Verlag, 1992), pp. 97–
98; Joel Richman, *Medicine and Health* (London: Longman, 1987), p. 10.

60. Richman, *Medicine and Health*, 10–11.

61. Julius Moravcsik, "Ancient and Modern Conceptions of Health and
Medicine," *Journal of Medicine and Philosophy* 1 (1976): 342.

62. The physician decides what is a symptom and who is sick. He
[or she] is a moral entrepreneur, charged with inquisitorial powers to
discover certain wrongs to be righted. Medicine, like all crusades, creates
a new group of outsiders each time it makes a new diagnosis stick.
Morality is as implicit in sickness as it is in crime or in sin.

Illich, *Limits of Medicine*, 54. Masturbation and menopause offer two examples
of conditions that have been transformed from the realm of the normal to
the realm of the diseased or vice versa. A hundred years ago, physicians
wrote of masturbation as an illness leading to general debility that was cured
by calming the nerves, hard work, tonics, sedatives, narcotics, restraining
devices, circumcision (of males and females), and other intrusive procedures.
Peter E.S. Freund and Meredith B. McGuire, *Health, Illness, and the Social Body:
A Critical Sociology* (Englewood Cliffs, N.J.: Prentice Hall, 1991), pp. 206–7.
Masturbation is no longer viewed as a disease and, in fact, is considered to
be normal. Ibid., 207. Menopause was, up to the last half century, understood
as simply a normal part of aging. Ibid., 209. Today, however, it is a deficiency
disease that is treatable through estrogen supplements. Ibid., 210.

63. Illich, *Limits to Medicine*, 54.

64. Freund, *Health, Illness, and the Social Body*, 6–7, 217–18.

65. Ibid. Consider the following statement about susceptibility to cancer: "Recent research shows cancer is not primarily caused by poisons spewed
out by uncaring industry. Rather, the villain appears to be an individual's
own genetic susceptibilities." "Genetic signposts on road to cancer," 8(D).
See also Illich, who writes:

[Medicine] serves to legitimize social arrangements into which many
people do not fit. It labels the handicapped as unfit and breeds ever
new categories of patients. People who are angered, sickened, and
impaired by their industrial labour and leisure can escape only into a
life under medical supervision and are thereby seduced or disqualified
from political struggle for a healthier world.

Illich, *Limits of Medicine*, 51.

66. Freund, *Health, Illness, and the Social Body*, 218.

67. Ibid. Alternatively, we find the cause for the individual's obesity in her or his genes. See Stephen Strauss, "Research team pinpoints gene that causes obesity," *(Toronto) Globe and Mail*, 1 December 1994, p. 1(A).

68. Freund, *Health, Illness, and the Social Body*, 232; Irving K. Zola, *Socio-Medical Inquiries: Recollections, Reflections, and Reconsiderations* (Philadelphia: Temple University Press, 1983), p. 219.

69. Freund, *Health, Illness, and the Social Body*, 233–34.

70. Zola, *Socio-Medical Inquiries*, 220.

71. Freund, *Health, Illness, and the Social Body*, 240, 243–44.

72. Ibid., 221, 225, 245.

73. Ibid., 255.

74. Richman, *Medicine and Health*, 20–21; Zola, *Socio-Medical Inquiries*, 86–108; Illich, *Limits to Medicine*, 134; Meredith B. McGuire, "Health and Spirituality as Contemporary Concerns," *Annals AAPSS* 527 (1993): 146; Margaret Read, *Culture, Health, and Disease* (London, Engl.: Tavistock Publications, 1966), p. 24.

75. See, e.g., Will Wright, *The Social Logic of Health* (New Brunswick, N.J.: Rutgers University Press, 1982), pp. 112–13.

76. Freund, *Health, Illness, and the Social Body*, 182–83, 185.

77. See Walzer, *Spheres of Justice*, 90.

78. Paul Tillich, "The Relation of Religion and Health," in *The Meaning of Health: Essays in Existentialism, Psychoanalysis, and Religion*, ed. Perry LeFevre (Chicago: Exploration Press, 1984), p. 17.

79. Ibid., 19; Matt. 11:5.

80. Tillich, "Relation of Religion and Health," 18–19.

81. Labisch, "Social Construction of Health," 86; Patrick J. Gallacher, "The *Summoner's Tale* and Medieval Attitudes Towards Sickness," *Chaucer Review* 21 (1986): 208.

82. David Kunzle, "The Art of Pulling Teeth in the Seventeenth and Nineteenth Centuries: From Public Martyrdom to Private Nightmare and Political Struggle?," in *Fragments for a History of the Human Body*, ed. Michel Feher (New York: Zone, 1989), p. 29.

83. See discussion chapter 7, n. 62.

84. Oscar Wilde, *The Picture of Dorian Gray* (New York: Illustrated Editions Co., 1931).

85. McGuire, "Health and Spirituality," 151–52.

86. Ibid., 145, 148–49, 154.

87. Freund, *Health, Illness, and the Social Body*, 6–7, 217.

88. 51 Cal. 3d 120 (1990).

89. See Kolata, "Biologist's Speedy Gene Method," 5(B).

90. Ribonucleic acid.

91. See Kolata, "Biologist's Speedy Gene Method" for a description of cDNA.

92. See ibid.

93. Strauss, "Research team pinpoints gene"; Ankney, "What if violent types are born," 20(A); Hess, "How the mating game evolved," 12(A).

94. Scott, *The Body as Property*, 1, 82–83.

95. Margaret J. Radin, "Justice in the Market Domain," in *NOMOS XXXI: Markets and Justice*, ed. John W. Chapman and J. Roland Pennock (New York: New York University Press, 1989), p. 169.

CHAPTER 8 NOTES

1. The laws of Æthelberht, ch. 53–54 (early seventh century) reprinted and translated in *The Laws of the Earliest English Kings*, ed. and trans. F.L. Attenborough (Cambridge: Cambridge University Press, 1922), p. 11.

2. 447 U.S. 303 (1980).

3. 631 F.2d 1264 (6th Cir. 1980).

4. If the current holder of the good is the person willing to pay the most for it, then she or he will retain it.

5. I choose this example because, while most of us take color perception for granted, it is far from straightforward.

6. The color superscale bears the same relationship to color as a meta-language of value bears to values. James Griffin's suggestion that "value" can be ranked on a scale of "well-being," which he argues makes values commensurable—James Griffin, *Well-Being: Its Meaning, Measurement, and Moral Importance* (Oxford: Oxford University Press, 1986), pp. 89–90—is analogous to the claim that color can be ranked on a color superscale. In neither case, as Griffin points out, is there any recourse to a "supervalue." Ibid., 89. That is, the color superscale and the scale of well-being do not measure substantive units of "color" or of "well-being;" rather, the color superscale ranks colors according to a particular—and, as stated in the text, artificial— conception of colorfulness, while the scale of well-being ranks values according to their contribution to a particular notion of well-being.

7. See Dennett, *Consciousness Explained*, 375.

8. Our determination of color is not perfect, however. That is why we often take objects, particularly clothing, into sunlight to determine their "real" color.

9. Michael Stocker, *Plural and Conflicting Values* (Oxford.: Clarendon Press, 1990), p. 198.

10. Anderson, *Value in Ethics and Economics*, p. 48. See also Hahnel & Albert, *Quiet Revolution in Welfare Economics*, 75–109; Taylor, *Sources of the Self*, 46–52.

11. Anderson, *Value in Ethics and Economics*, p. 60.

12. Nussbaum, *The Fragility of Goodness*, 295.

13. Griffin, *Well-Being*, 89.

14. It is not clear where Gillian ranks autonomy, since either choice implicates autonomy, albeit in different ways.

15. See Taylor, *Sources of the Self*, 47; Dennett, *Consciousness Explained*, 410; Nussbaum, *The Fragility of Goodness*, 306.

16. Joseph Raz, *The Morality of Freedom* (Oxford: Clarendon Press, 1986), p. 325.

17. Anderson, *Value in Ethics and Economics*, pp. 58, 70.

18. Ibid., p. 51.

19. Raz, *The Morality of Freedom*, 339.

20. Ibid.; Stocker, *Plural and Conflicting Values*, 198.

21. Anderson, *Value in Ethics and Economics*, p. 47.

22. 51 Cal. 3d 120 (1990).

23. It further ignores the fact that, despite highly interventionist and reductionalist techniques in medical care, the practice of medicine—as opposed to better nutrition, better sanitation, and other public health measures—has contributed only slightly to the increase in the life span of individuals in the United States. Freund, *Health, Illness, and the Social Body*, 20.

24. For example, the choice to abort those fetuses with the genetic potential to get Huntington's disease or diabetes.

25. Stocker, *Plural and Conflicting Values*, 154.

26. 631 F.2d 1264 (6th Cir. 1980).

CHAPTER 9 NOTES

1. Italo Calvino, "The Dinosaurs," in *Cosmicomics*, trans. William Weaver (New York: Harcourt Brace Jovanovich, 1968), pp. 111–12.

2. U.S. Const. amend. XIII. See also, U.S. Const. amend. XIV and XV.

3. See, e.g., Brown v. Board of Educ., 347 U.S. 483 (1954).

4. See, e.g., Swann v. Charlotte-Mecklenberg Bd. of Educ., 402 U.S. 1 (1971).

5. 447 U.S. 303 (1980).

6. See discussion pp. 82–83.

7. In the discussion in chapter 8 regarding how in Local 1330, United Steel Workers of America v. United States Steel Corp., 631 F.2d 1264 (6th Cir. 1980) the court could have dealt with noneconomic values inhering in steel mills through other branches of the law. I deferred discussion of this strategy until this chapter.

8. Radin, "Property and Personhood," 957, 972–73. Waldron, *The Right of Private Property*, similarly puts forth a self-development rationale for property.

9. Hegel, *Philosophy of Right*.

10. Radin, "Property and Personhood," 986.

11. William H. Simon, "Social-Republican Property," *University of California at Los Angeles Law Review* 38 (1991): 1340–41.

12. Laura S. Underkuffler, "On Property," *Yale Law Journal* 100 (1990): 138, 141–42.

13. Ibid., 139. See also Diana Belevsky, "Liberty as Property," *University of Toronto Law Journal* 45 (1995): 209.

14. Underkuffler, "On Property," 139–40, 143–44.

15. Posner, *The Economics of Justice*, 69–72.

16. In addition to these theorists, others suggest different modes of valuing goods. For example, Singer, "The Reliance Interest in Property," argues that, through property, goods ought to be valued in terms of sharing. Stephen R. Munzer, *A Theory of Property* (Cambridge: Cambridge University Press, 1990) suggests that property rights rest upon a plurality of reasons, including utilitarian considerations, Kantian or Rawlsian considerations of justice, and considerations of desert. Therefore, Munzer's conception of property promotes a mixture of several modes of valuing goods. Still other theorists argue that property has become a meaningless concept. Thomas C. Grey, "The Disintegration of Property," in *NOMOS XXII: Property*, ed. J. Roland Pennock and John W. Chapman (New York: New York University Press, 1980), p. 69.

17. See Gold, "A Structural Dynamic Theory of Law," 347 for a more detailed discussion of the process of change within law.

18. Hannah Arendt, *The Human Condition* (Chicago: University of Chicago Press, 1958).

19. Ibid.

20. Taylor, *Sources of the Self*, 26.

21. Michael Albert et al., *Liberating Theory* (Boston.: South End Press, 1986), p. 20.

22. Dennett, *Consciousness Explained*, 416; Arendt, *The Human Condition*, 179–80.

23. White, *Justice as Translation*, 50.

24. Dennett, *Consciousness Explained*, 417.

25. See Jane E. Brody, "For Snow the Real Action Begins After It Falls," *New York Times*, 9 February 1988, p. 1(C). But see Steven Pinker, *The Language Instinct* (New York: HarperCollins, 1994), pp. 64–65.

26. Certainly former Vice President Dan Quayle does not seem able to envision that a single woman with a child is a "family." See, e.g., Andrew Rosenthal, "Quayle Says Riots Arose from Burst of Social Anarchy," *New York Times*, 20 May 1992, pp. 1(A), 11(A); "Excerpts From Vice President's Speech on Cities and Poverty," *New York Times*, 20 May 1992, p. 11(A); Michael Wines, "Appeal of 'Murphy Brown' Now Clear at White House," *New York Times*, 21 May 1992, pp. 1(A), 12(A).

27. Although he does not specifically state that reification occurs partly through language, György Lukács, *History and Class Consciousness: Studies in Marxist Dialectics*, trans. Rodney Livingstone (Cambridge, Mass.: MIT Press, 1971), pp. 93, 100 posits that the manner in which we act, specifically by market exchange, fundamentally shapes our understanding of the world. See also Gold, "Structural Dynamic Theory of Law," for a discussion of how ideology becomes reified in the language of the law.

28. Zola, "Healthism and Disabling Medicalization," 64. See also Lippman, "Prenatal Genetic Testing and Screening," 24:

Prenatal diagnosis presupposes that certain fetal conditions are intrinsically not bearable. Increasing diagnostic capability means that such conditions, as well as a host of variations that can be detected *in utero*, are proliferating, necessarily broadening the range of what is not "bearable" and restricting concepts of what is "normal." It is, perhaps, not unreasonable to ask if the "imperfect" will become anything we can diagnose.

29. See David B. Wilkins, "Presumed Crazy: The Structure of Argument in the Hill/Thomas Hearings," *Southern California Law Review* 65 (1992): 1517.

30. See Zola, "Healthism and Disabling Medicalization," 63.

31. White, *Justice as Translation*, 50.

32. Margaret Radin would go further than is required here, and argue that discussing a good in terms of its economic value actually degrades our appreciation of that good:

> Market rhetoric, if adopted by everyone, and in many contexts, would indeed transform the texture of the human world. This rhetoric leads us to view politics as just rent seeking, reproductive capacity as just a scarce good for which there is high demand, and the repugnance of slavery as just a cost. To accept these views is to accept the conception of human flourishing they imply, one that is inferior to the conception we can accept as properly ours. An inferior conception of human flourishing disables us from conceptualizing the world rightly. Market rhetoric, the rhetoric of alienability of all "goods," is also the rhetoric of alienation of ourselves from what we can be as persons.

Margaret J. Radin, "Market-Inalienability," *Harvard Law Review* 100, (1987): 1884–85.

33. White, *Justice as Translation*, 57–58.

34. Radin, "Market-Inalienability," 1877–84.

35. Gold, "Structural Dynamic Theory of Law," 366–68, 371–73.

36. *See* Vandevelde, "New Property of the Nineteenth Century;" Charles Donahue, Jr., "The Future of the Concept of Property Predicated from its Past," in *Nomos XXII: Property*, ed. J. Roland Pennock and John W. Chapman (New York: New York University Press, 1980), p. 28; Horwitz, *The Transformation of American Law*. Although Horwitz's book has been criticized on several fronts, his basic thesis that the conception of property within the law changed in the nineteenth century seems to have been generally accepted. See, e.g., Robert J. Gordon, "Critical Legal Histories," *Stanford Law Review* 36 (1984): 96–97; Jennifer Nedelsky, *Private Property and the Limits of American Constitutionalism: The Madisonian Framework and Its Legacy* (Chicago: University of Chicago Press, 1990), p. 319. But see Alan Watson, "The Transformation of American Property Law: A Comparative Law Approach," *Georgia Law Review* 24 (1990): 186–216.

37. As the spirit of economic development began to take hold of American society in the early years of the nineteenth century, however, the idea of property underwent a fundamental transformation—from a static agrarian conception entitling an owner to undisturbed enjoyment, to a dynamic, instrumental, and more abstract view of property that emphasized the newly paramount virtues of use and development.

Horwitz, *The Transformation of American Law*, 31.

38. Nedelsky, *Private Property*, 243.

39. Radin, "Property and Personhood," 994.

40. Radin, "Market-Inalienability," 1932–34.

41. See, e.g., Wesley N. Hohfeld, "Some Fundamental Legal Conceptions as Applied to Judicial Reasoning," *Yale Law Journal* 23 (1913): 45 n.67; Honoré, "Ownership," 113; C.B. Macpherson, "Human Rights as Property Rights," in *The Rise and Fall of Economic Justice and Other Papers* (Oxford: Oxford University Press, 1985) p. 81.

42. Armstrong, "The Reification of Celebrity," 443.

43. See U.S. Const. amend. V.

44. Jennifer Nedelsky, "American Constitutionalism and the Paradox of Private Property," in *Constitutionalism and Democracy: Studies in Rationality and Social Change*, ed. Jon Elster and Rune Slagstad (Cambridge: Cambridge University Press, 1988), p. 252 n.

45. Honoré, "Ownership," 114 states that:

The protection of the right to possess, and so of one essential element in ownership, is achieved only when there are rules allocating exclusive physical control to one person rather than another, and that not merely on the basis that the person who has such control at the moment is entitled to continue in control.

46. 433 U.S. 562 (1976).

47. Waldron, *The Right to Private Property*, 39 states that "[t]he owner of a resource is simply the individual whose determination as to the use of the resource is taken as final in a system [of private property]."

48. 51 Cal. 3d 120 (1990).

49. One can share Margaret Radin's hope, expressed in Margaret J. Radin, "The Consequences of Conceptualism," *University of Miami Law Review* 41 (1986): 243, that property discourse will change over time to include such other modes of evaluation, without agreeing that it is appropriate now to subject the human body to this discourse. Contra Nedelsky, *Private Property*, 253.

Index

Abel, 132

algorithm, 70; patentability of, 72, 75

altruism, 142, 156

Aquinas, Thomas: body of, 131

Arabian, Justice, 35–39

Arendt, Hannah, 169

Aristotle, 210n.47

artistic integrity: modes of valuing, 113–14

autonomy, 139, 144–45, 156

Benson. See *Gottschalk v. Benson*

biotechnology, 1–2, 19, 64, 80, 168; definition of, 179n.2; non-human 66, 78

blood, 131, 185–86n.51; boiling, 132; modes of valuing, 12, 13; relationship to health, 13; as speaking of cause of death, 132

body, 174; application of property discourse to, 17; as boundary, 129; as commodity, 2; components of, 2, 13–14; and culture, 128; decisions regarding, 4; as reflection of divine, 132; and equality, 128; female, 133; gifts of, 131; and identity, 129, 130; male, 127, 133; marking of, 126, 128, 133; modes of valuing, 1, 5, 12, 17, 21, 130, 147; photographs of, 131; and property, 161; as po-

litical metaphor, 127; reductionalism with respect to, 128; relics from, 131; and ritual, 130; as sacred good, 2; and sex, 133; and sin, 132, 133; and soul, 130; and will, 130

body parts. *See* human biological materials

Brandeis, Justice, 56, 59–60

Broussard, Justice, 28–31

Cain, 133

Camus, Albert, 135

cancer, 211n.65

capital punishment 134–35

Carson v. Here's Johnny Portable Toilets, 102–3

cell-line, 138–39

Chakrabarty. See *Diamond v. Chakrabarty*

color: commensurability of, 149, 151; perception of, 151; scale of, 149, 152

commensurability: of color, 151; distinguished from comparison, 158; and property discourse, 22; and ranking modes of valuation, 11; and super-scale of value, 153; of value, 9, 11, 17, 21, 32, 47, 61, 147, 149, 154–55, 157–59, 161

commodification, 38, 175